A Han

Traine

A Handbook for Trainee Psychiatrists

Edited by

KEITH J. B. RIX
BMedBiol, MPhil, MD, CBiol, MIBiol, MRCPsych

Senior Lecturer in Psychiatry, University of Leeds, Consultant Psychiatrist, St James's University Hospital, Leeds

Baillière Tindall London Philadelphia
Toronto Sydney Tokyo

Baillière Tindall
W. B. Saunders

24–28 Oval Road
London NW1 7DX, England

West Washington Square
Philadelphia, PA 19105, USA

1 Goldthorne Avenue
Toronto, Ontario M8Z 5T9, Canada

ABP Australia Ltd, 44 Waterloo Road
North Ryde, NSW 2064, Australia

Harcourt Brace Jovanovich Japan Inc.
Ichibancho Central Building, 22–1 Ichibancho
Chiyoda-ku, Tokyo 102, Japan

First published 1987

Printed and bound in Great Britain by
The Guernsey Press Co. Ltd., Guernsey, Channel Islands.

British Library Cataloguing in Publication Data

A handbook for trainee psychiatrists.
1. Psychiatry
I. Rix, Keith J.B.
616.89 RC454

ISBN 0 7020 1199 1

Contents

Section 2 Aspects of Treatment

Section 3 Special Topics

Contributors

Francis Creed, MA, MD, MRCP, MRCPsych, Senior Lecturer in Psychiatry, University of Manchester.

J. F. W. Deakin, MB, ChB, PhD, MRCPsych, Senior Lecturer in Psychiatry, University of Manchester.

Graham Glancy, MB, ChB, MRCPsych, FRCP(C), Assistant Professor of Psychiatry, University of Toronto and Staff Psychiatrist, Clarke Institute, Toronto.

David Goldberg, MA, MSc, DM, FRCP, FRCPsych, Professor of Psychiatry, University of Manchester.

Maurice Greenberg, MB, MPhil, Dip Biochem, MRCP, MRCPsych, Consultant Psychiatrist, Jules Thorn Psychiatric Day Hospital, St Pancras Hospital, London.

Tim Jerram, BA, MB, BCh, MRCPI, MRCPsych, Lecturer in Psychiatry, University of Leeds and Consultant Psychiatrist, High Royds Hospital, Menston, Ilkley, West Yorkshire.

T. Kay, MB, ChB, DMJ, MRCPsych, Consultant Forensic Psychiatrist, Newton Lodge, Wakefield.

P. J. McKenna, BA, MB, ChB, MRCPsych, Lecturer in Psychiatry, University of Leeds.

Peter Maguire, MA, MB, BChir, MRCPsych, Senior Lecturer in Psychiatry, University of Manchester.

Frank Margison, MB, ChB, MSc, MRCPsych, Consultant Psychotherapist, Manchester Royal Infirmary.

R. H. S. Mindham, MD, DCH, FRCP(Ed), FRCPsych, Nuffield Professor of Psychiatry, University of Leeds.

I. Pennell, MB, ChB, MSc, MRCPsych, Research Fellow, Department of Psychiatry, University of Manchester.

Philip H. Rack, MA, MB, BChir, FRCPsych, Consultant Psychiatrist, Lynfield Mount Hospital, Bradford.

Keith J. B. Rix, BMedBiol, MPhil, MD, CBiol, MIBiol, MRCPsych, Senior Lecturer in Psychiatry, University of Leeds and Consultant Psychiatrist, St James's University Hospital, Leeds.

Andrew Sims, MA, MD, FRCPsych, Professor of Psychiatry, University of Leeds.

R. P. Snaith, MD, FRCPsych, Senior Lecturer in Psychiatry, University of Leeds.

David Storer, MB, ChB, MRCPsych, Lecturer in Psychiatry, University of Leeds and Consultant Psychiatrist, Leeds General Infirmary.

E. Szabadi, MD, PhD, DSc, Dip Neurol, FRCPsych, Reader in Psychiatry, University of Manchester.

Digby Tantam, MB, ChB, MPH, MRCPsych, Senior Lecturer in Psychiatry, University of Manchester.

J. P. Wattis, MB, ChB, MRCPsych, Consultant Psychiatrist, St James's University Hospital, Leeds.

Foreword

By Thomas Bewley
President of the Royal College of Psychiatrists

The Royal College of Psychiatrists is enjoined by its charter to improve standards of care and treatment in psychiatry, which includes promoting the education and training of psychiatrists. Although medicine is science-based all branches of it retain some elements of craft and art. Junior psychiatrists, and those colleagues in other branches of medicine who also require training in psychiatry, need psychiatric textbooks and journals. They also need other practical information that may be found in a syllabus or in examination regulations or that given in the *Handbook for Inceptors* that was produced by the College. There is a gulf between these two types of publication and it is one that Dr Keith Rix and his colleagues have endeavoured to fill in this new handbook for trainee psychiatrists. Although its aim is to give very practical instruction to the most junior of psychiatrists, nevertheless there is much in it which will be useful to more senior colleagues and psychiatric tutors. Dr Szabadi, for example, spells out very clearly eight different reasons that make it necessary for psychiatrists to examine their patients physically, a point that is not always covered so thoroughly. The contributors, generally, work in Leeds and in Manchester and it is good that their sensible advice will now be available to trainees in other parts of the country. Books of this type are usually slated by reviewers when they first appear on the grounds that they are sordid, unduly practical manuals and thus anti-educational. However, a book such as this, which is well written, soundly based and provides useful advice, soon establishes its worth and is widely read. I will be interested to follow its progress.

Thomas H. Bewley, MA, MD, FRCPI, FRCPsych

Preface

After a year of medical and surgical house jobs the psychiatry clerkship is likely to be recalled even less distinctly than it was at final MB examinations. Without your white coat and surrounded by a multidisciplinary team you may feel a little unsure of yourself. For all your good intentions of practising holistic medicine when you started house jobs, the plain fact is that you cannot remember how to take the sort of psychiatric history and carry out the sort of mental state examination which will be expected of you in a psychiatry training post. Furthermore, if you intend obtaining Membership of the Royal College of Psychiatrists you will have to demonstrate a certain level of clinical skill in the new Part 1 examination, which is usually taken after a year of psychiatric training. Although some of the earlier chapters in this book may appear to cover 'bread and butter' subjects mastered at the undergraduate level, this may be just the sort of initial diet necessary to achieve fitness for the Part 1.

How you use this book will depend on your stage of training and needs. If you are a medical student or houseman thinking about applying for a psychiatry post you might start with Chapter 1 (Making the Most of a Rotational Training Scheme) and perhaps Chapter 2 (Responsibilities of the Junior Psychiatric Trainee). As a newly appointed senior house officer you could usefully start with Chapter 2 and read through to Chapter 10 the night before starting the job. Once in post you should read the chapters on treatment (Chapters 11 to 14) fairly soon if you have not already done so. The rest of the chapters do not need to be read quite so soon and some can be left until a particular situation arises. However, it is never too early to read about studying, examinations and research. The final chapter (A North American

Perspective) may be of interest if you are thinking of going to North America as well as being important if you are a North American reader who wants to see the rest of the chapters in the context of North American psychiatric practice. Since some trainees will want to read chapters in isolation, overlap between chapters has not been completely eliminated.

Keith J. B. Rix

Acknowledgements

I am grateful to Frank Margison for contributing the psychodynamic psychopathology entries for the glossary. The rest of the glossary is based on an earlier version which I prepared with Christopher Fairburn (now of the University of Oxford). Since we have both been PSE-trained our definitions of descriptive psychopathological terms have been considerably influenced by the approach to descriptive psychopathology in the Present State Examination (J. K. Wing, J. E. Cooper and N. Sartorius, *Measurement and Classification of Psychiatric Symptoms,* Cambridge University Press, 1974).

Bob Holt and Stephen Jones kindly gave me the benefit of their legal knowledge in relation to Chapter 16 and Drs Jo Banbery, J. Cunnane, Sue Jones and D. Tombs criticized drafts of various chapters.

I am also grateful to Nick Dunton and David Cross of Baillière Tindall for their help in producing this book.

Keith J. B. Rix

Section 1
Working as a Junior Psychiatrist

— 1 —

Making the Most of a Rotational Training Scheme

David Storer

APPLYING FOR A PLACE

When a vacancy occurs in a popular training scheme 50–100 applications may be received. It is clearly important to be able to show some extra enthusiasm or ability for psychiatry even to be short-listed. Having obtained a distinction in psychiatry or carried out an elective period in the specialty will obviously help. Interesting activities and accomplishments outside medicine may be useful too, but somehow all applicants seem to play two or three musical instruments and to be marathon runners.

Applicants should, if possible, try and talk to at least the psychiatric tutor (often called 'clinical tutor') before the interview. Knowing one of the other consultants or trainees may help the applicant to find out more about the scheme and what is being looked for in potential trainees. There are, of course, rules against canvassing but most consultants appreciate a reasonable attempt on behalf of potential applicants to find out what they are applying for. Psychiatric tutors are frequently not given adequate time to carry out their duties and he or she will not be able to see all of the applicants over a short period. In this case, only those short-listed may be invited to visit so your typewritten application is very important. There is nothing to stop an interested applicant writing to the psychiatric tutor before an advertisement appears, seeking general advice and information. The tutor may be more easily able to find time to see the applicant away from the usual advertising time.

Once an applicant is short-listed his chances of being accepted will depend, to a great extent, on his performance at interview. This is perhaps regrettable to some extent as it is his clinical ability with patients which should count, not his ability to impress at a short interview. However, it is sensible to reduce the likelihood of creating an unfavourable impression. Unfortunately, interview committees as well as candidates have their idiosyncrasies but the usual advice of dressing smartly but not flashily and at least being polite to the interviewers does have some validity. It is certainly going to count against an applicant if he does not appear to care whether he wants the place or not but candidates who over-do this can make the committee wonder why they are so desperate for a job.

The candidate will at some point be asked if he has any questions. If he has done his research well beforehand it is quite reasonable to say that he has none to ask, but if there are still some points on which clarification is needed, he should ask at this point. Should the candidate be offered a place it is likely that he will have to accept there and then so he should make sure that he has no serious doubts.

PLACEMENTS

Trainees may or may not be given a choice of first post in the scheme; this will depend on how the scheme is organized. If there is a choice it is sensible to start in general psychiatry if possible. In many schemes the psychiatrists for the elderly take all patients aged over 65 years so these posts can also be regarded as good starting places.

In most schemes the trainee is able to have at least some influence on the units or teams to which he will be attached. It is important to complete, during the length of the scheme, a good range of attachments. At least a total of one year should be spent in general psychiatry although such specialties as rehabilitation, liaison psychiatry and psychiatry of old age do have a substantial component of general psychiatry. The usual length of a placement is six months but there is something to be said for spending a longer period in one post in general psychiatry, perhaps at the beginning of the scheme. This allows the trainee to get more of a feel of the way in which a team operates and to see patients over a longer period than usual. Some schemes include shorter placements in specialties such as mental handicap or forensic psychiatry, which can be valuable. An alternative to shorter placements is a system of part-time attachments; this system may work but has the disadvantage that the trainee can feel something of an outsider in both units compared to full-time staff. The trainee will gain a fair idea of which of the placements available will particularly suit him from discussing them with colleagues who have already done that placement. Points to ask about include:

Amount of clinical work

If a unit is so busy that there is insufficient time for each patient then the trainee will learn less than if he is able to devote a reasonable length of time to each case. On the other hand, a post in which there is not enough clinical material is even worse.

Adequate supervision and appropriate level of responsibility

A great deal can be learned from patients but the experience is so much more valuable if the trainee can discuss cases with someone more experienced. Ward rounds can be an invaluable teaching exercise but on some units they are merely 'business' occasions to make decisions about drug treatment, discharge, weekend leave, etc., and this reduces their value considerably to the trainee. Out-patient clinics are often the best experience for the trainee as they provide one to one contact with patients over a long period. It is important, however, that the trainee is not left alone to make unsupervised decisions. A consultant or senior registrar should be available, preferably in the clinic, for advice. The trainee should be given scope to make decisions and manage problems himself, but there should be regular supervision sessions.

Medical colleagues

A large team is not necessarily better than a 'firm' of one consultant and one trainee. The close 'apprenticeship' relationship the latter can produce can be a particularly valuable learning experience. Working for more than one consultant at a time can present problems even though it may be unavoidable in some units.

Non-medical colleagues

Probably in psychiatry more than any other specialty, being able to work with non-medical colleagues is an essential part of your training. Being able to choose placements in teams which operate in a genuinely multidisciplinary way will add considerably to the learning opportunities (see Chapter 3).

When asked to express preferences for specialist posts there are also particular points to look out for, which vary from specialty to specialty:

General psychiatry

A placement should offer supervised in-patient and out-patient work. If the scheme is in an area which still has long-stay wards then such experience should not be regarded as a drawback in a placement. A great deal can be learned from these chronic, perhaps institutionalized, patients. However, the balance should not be so far towards long-stay care that the trainee spends a high proportion of time dealing with the physical problems of a large population of hospital residents. It is also important to work with day patients. This may be as part of a general placement or there may be a specialized day hospital attachment on the scheme. It should be an active unit, not one where only a long-term population of schizophrenics visit daily in the absence of other provision.

Alcohol and drug dependence

This may be a full-time placement or with a consultant who has a 'special responsibility' or 'special interest'. It is unlikely that there will be a choice between units on any one scheme. Before opting for such a placement the trainee should be prepared to work in a fairly close relationship, either on an individual or group basis, with often difficult patients and also with non-medical personnel who will be considerably more familiar with the techniques involved than he can be in a relatively short attachment.

Child and adolescent psychiatry

Child and adolescent psychiatry is an important branch of the specialty in which to gain some experience. Most child psychiatrists operate very differently from adult psychiatrists and it is an approach which needs to be experienced. Trainees who have not worked in child psychiatry will not know whether it would appeal to them as a career. However, many schemes cannot offer a placement in a child and adolescent unit to all trainees.

Forensic psychiatry

Most forensic units offer training mainly at senior registrar level. Think carefully before volunteering to work in this area early in your training.

Consultation-liaison psychiatry

This can be a rewarding specialty in which to work, particularly for trainees who enjoy contact with non-psychiatric medical colleagues. Most schemes in non-teaching hospitals will not have a specific attachment. If one does exist make sure it is not merely a question of nominating one trainee to see all the self-poisoning cases although some units offering full-time work in the assessment of deliberate self-harm can offer extremely valuable and interesting training. If it is necessary to see self-poisoning cases, make sure supervision and teaching are available so that it does not become merely a difficult chore.

Mental handicap

All psychiatrists have, at least from time to time, to deal with mentally handicapped patients and it is increasingly common for joint appointments between general psychiatry and mental handicap to be advertised at consultant level. Most mental handicap units are keen to take on general psychiatric trainees for short periods and offer good educational attachments. Beware the minority who use registrars largely to look after the physical needs of large numbers of long-stay residents.

Psychiatry of old age

Psychogeriatrics is an expanding branch of psychiatry. An enthusiastic multidisciplinary psychogeriatric team actively involved in the community can be one of the most enjoyable and stimulating placements but make sure, in psychiatry of the elderly even more than other specialties, that there is regular involvement in domiciliary visits, visits to community facilities and in working with psychiatric community nurses.

Psychotherapy

Individual and group psychotherapy needs to be experienced over longer periods than the normal six-month attachment. If there is a specific attachment in the scheme clarify the arrangements for being able to follow patients through after the attachment ends. Try to ensure at least one placement with a unit where behavioural treatments are used.

Rehabilitation

If an attachment in rehabilitation is available it should be in a unit with reasonable facilities and a good throughput of patients. Sometimes the rehabilitation consultant is saddled with the most difficult patients that no-one else wants and, paradoxically, may have the lowest turnover. While these patients can provide interesting and valuable experience an active unit can provide more training in rehabilitation techniques. This is another part of psychiatry where it is particularly important to see facilities available outside of hospital.

Once allocated to a particular post the trainee should try to establish the expectations a consultant has of him as soon as possible. Conversely, he may feel able to discuss with the consultant his own training needs from the posts as he sees them. Ideally, the relationship with the consultant should be one where progress is reviewed on an on-going basis. However, some consultants are reticent to discuss this and the trainee should ask for at least a mid-placement discussion in which both the consultant and himself can look at the way in which the placement is fulfilling his needs and what his weaknesses may be. This then allows the second half of the placement for improving matters. Some schemes have a formal review built into the system for this purpose.

PSYCHIATRIC TUTORS

Some schemes will be administered by one psychiatric tutor. Larger ones may be organized by several tutors working together, while others may have an organizing committee usually chaired by one of the psychiatric tutors.

The psychiatric tutor at hospital level will have the responsibility to ensure case conferences, journal clubs and other meetings are organized. In addition, he should monitor and review the progress of trainees through the scheme. While a trainee would normally approach his or her own consultant on most matters, the tutor should provide continuity throughout the period of the scheme. Any problem relating to training should be taken to the psychiatric tutor by the trainee. A tutor should also be seen as the trainees' advocate and supporter in committees.

Tutors may or may not be recognized by the local university or by the various NHS committees but all must be recognized by the Royal College of Psychiatrists.

The College lays down guidelines governing the role and duties of tutors. These include the regular discussion of progress with the trainees. The trainee may find that his tutor meets regularly with trainees as a group or on an individual basis or both.

The tutor will be trying to combine the somewhat difficult and time-consuming duties of a psychiatric tutor with what will, almost certainly, be a busy consultant job. He should be allocated two sessions per week to do this but quite possibly these sessions will be somewhat nominal. If a trainee feels that his tutor is not fulfilling all of the duties of his post as well as he should then he may well be aware of this but be unable to devote more time to do so. However, if a view that the tutor is not carrying out his role satisfactorily is shared by most of the trainees then this should be discussed if possible with the tutor himself but, if not, with the other consultant staff. This is obviously somewhat difficult for trainees but when the College approval visit takes place the role of the tutor in a hospital will be carefully examined and it is better if difficulties have been aired and hopefully resolved before then. Most psychiatric tutors are only too aware of the imperfections in their own scheme and are grateful for the opportunity to constructively discuss ways in which things can be improved.

One of the less well-defined roles of the tutor is to be available to discuss any personal difficulties the trainee may have. This does not mean that the tutor will wish to pry into a trainee's personal life. A trainee who wishes to discuss personal difficulties will know who he feels able to talk to about this – it may or may not be the tutor.

However, psychiatry can be more stressful to some doctors than other branches of medicine and psychiatric patients can often make demands which an inexperienced doctor may find difficult. Some forms of psychotherapy, in particular, actually use the patient's emotional feelings towards the therapist as a therapeutic tool. If carrying out psychotherapy, skilled supervision is essential and the trainee will find this a help in dealing with such problems (see Chapter 11). Outside of formal psychotherapy he may find similar problems and while his own consultant should offer help with this, he may turn to the psychiatric tutor for additional support.

Some psychiatric trainees find personal therapy from a psychotherapist particularly helpful but this may be more fruitful at a later stage in training.

ORGANIZATION OF SCHEMES

There are basically two types of rotational training scheme. The first is the 'fixed' type where upon entry the trainee knows for the next three to four years which placements will be carried out. The second is the totally flexible organization where, at intervals, all or most of the trainees are moved around with varying degrees of trainee choice exercised.

Most schemes are based on some sort of compromise between these two extremes. Commonly, posts are allocated for the first year and then placements are made taking into account the training needs and desires of the trainees. Increasingly, promotion from SHO to registrar will be made more or less automatically, subject to satisfactory progress.

It is important to try to ensure as wide a variety of placements as possible. The College recommends as many as possible from a list including: (1) General Psychiatry, (2) Alcohol and

Drug Dependence, (3) Child and Adolescent Psychiatry, (4) Forensic Psychiatry, (5) Liaison Work, (6) Mental Handicap, (7) Psychiatry of Old Age, (8) Psychotherapy, (9) Rehabilitation.

Trainees in a scheme should organize themselves into a committee which should decide where to press for improvements in a training scheme and elect representatives to other committees including the local Division of Psychiatry. Many schemes have an organizing committee which will include trainee representatives although they will not usually be present when individual colleagues are being discussed.

THE APPROVAL EXERCISE

One of the responsibilities of the College is to ensure that the standard of training in psychiatry in the United Kingom and Ireland is maintained and improved. One of the key parts of this process is the approval exercise. The College recognizes training schemes as suitable for psychiatric training and periodically schemes are visited by an 'approval panel'. The panel consists of three psychiatrists, almost always including one trainee. By far the most valuable information to them is that given by trainees. Trainees whose scheme is visited should give an honest account of the strengths and weaknesses of the training as they see it.

MOVING ON

After completing three to four years' psychiatric training and obtaining the MRCPsych trainees will be looking towards the next stage in their training. For most people this will be a senior registrar (SR) post but some may be attracted by an academic (lecturer) post or by a full-time research appointment.

Most SR posts are in a general psychiatry rotation scheme

with placements in special interests but trainees who have decided to pursue a career in child psychiatry or psychotherapy are likely to look for a full-time post in that specialty. There is also an increasing number of full-time senior registrar posts in forensic psychiatry. Mental handicap has, in the past, had its own SR posts but there has recently been a movement towards integrating mental handicap with general psychiatry senior registrar schemes.

When deciding in which direction to move after the registrar post remember that the next job will be seen very clearly as preparing the way for a consultant post and the psychiatrist may well be thereafter in one post for the rest of his working life. Obviously, this is a time for very careful and clear thought about how to spend the rest of one's career.

The chances of a good post at SR level will be enhanced if the trainee has taken full advantage of a good rotational training scheme. If he can offer something else, such as an interesting research project (see Chapter 20), then he will be in an even stronger position.

Further reading

Royal College of Psychiatrists (1985) *Careers in Psychiatry*
Royal College of Psychiatrists (1986) *Hospitals, Units and Training Schemes Approved for General Professional Training*

2

Responsibilities of the Junior Psychiatric Trainee

Keith J. B. Rix

THE PSYCHIATRIC TEAM

The SHO or occasionally the registrar is the most junior medical member of a psychiatric team which is headed by a consultant. There may be another SHO or registrar (junior trainees) and there may be an SR (senior trainee) who acts for the consultant in his absence and provides some of the day-to-day supervision of the junior trainees. In teaching hospitals the consultant may be a university professor, reader, senior lecturer or lecturer with an honorary NHS contract. Similarly, in addition to or instead of the SR, there may be a university lecturer or tutor, or occasionally a research fellow, with an honorary NHS contract at the SR level.

If there is another SHO or registrar this is the person most likely to be able to explain what the post entails but, if the other junior trainee is also new, the SR is likely to be able to do this. Broadly speaking the responsibilities of the junior psychiatric trainee beginning his training in general psychiatry lie in the area of in-patients, out-patients and day patients. This chapter will concentrate on general psychiatry because it is in general psychiatry posts that most trainees will begin their training and by the time they rotate to sub-specialty posts they are less likely to need a handbook.

In addition to the medical staff the psychiatric trainee is likely to be working alongside nurses, social workers, occupational therapists, clinical psychologists and occasionally other professionals (Chapter 3).

IN-PATIENTS

Having ascertained on which wards there are in-patients for whom he is responsible, the junior trainee needs to either acquaint himself with the arrangements for discussing them on a daily basis or make such arrangements. Some patients will be fairly disturbed and on weekdays they need to be discussed daily by the doctors and nurses involved. Some teams have formal arrangements for a meeting, usually at the beginning of a working day, when all in-patients are discussed by nurses and their respective doctors. If such arrangements do not exist the trainee should make arrangements with the nurses to visit the ward at particular times. If study leave arrangements or other commitments prevent the trainee from visiting the ward on a particular day of the week, alternative arrangements should be made involving, for example, the other junior trainee or the SR. The nursing staff should be informed in advance.

The frequency with which the trainee sees individual patients is determined by their clinical state and treatment. Patients who continue to be disturbed and patients whose diagnosis is not yet clear should be seen on a daily basis in order to establish rapport, record their mental state, complete history taking and, if appropriate, make day-to-day adjustments in medication. Patients who have ECT ought to have a mental state examination between each application. Some patients whose treatment is largely psychotherapeutic and whose individual treatment is being carried out by the junior trainee need to be seen at specified times for a specified period of time.

Sometimes general psychiatric trainees have responsibility for one or more medium or long-stay (including psychogeriatric) wards. These wards should be visited at least once a week and arrangements made to ensure that all patients in turn are regularly reviewed at the ward rounds or team meetings. All patients should have a complete physical and mental state examination at least every six months.

CASE RECORDS

Several purposes are served by case records: they are a place in which to store information; they are a means of communication between different health professionals; they may be a source of information for clinical or epidemiological research; they constitute a document which may be produced in a court of law or other judicial tribunal when legal issues arise out of the patient's case.

As repositories of information it is important that information is stored according to some logical arrangement. Not all systems for filing documents in case records are as logical as they might be but it is important that the trainee familiarises himself with the local system and adheres strictly to it.

The value of case records in communications is also influenced by their legibility. There is no excuse for illegible case notes. Furthermore, communication is enhanced if all entries have a heading (e.g. Progress Note, Discussion with Relatives etc.), date and sometimes time, signature, the name if the signature is illegible, status of the person writing the note and the name of the responsible consultant.

If case records are any use in research not only must they be accurate but they must contain detailed descriptions of symptoms and signs as well as psychopathological labels and diagnostic conclusions. The importance of recording verbatim accounts of symptoms and observations rather than conclusions is discussed further in Chapter 6.

When considering the medicolegal status of case records it is important to consider not only accuracy, reliability and legibility but also the need to avoid the use of slang and pejorative terms which could cause the writer some embarrassment in a witness box and misleadingly call into question the reliability of his evidence. Errors should be deleted with a single line so that what was originally written is still legible.

Finally it should be remembered that case records belong

to the Secretary of State and are confidential, often intimately detailed, accounts of people's private lives. Their security and confidentiality must be respected.

WARD ROUNDS AND TEAM MEETINGS

Management of in-patients on acute wards will be mainly decided upon at a weekly or twice-weekly ward round or team meeting chaired usually by the consultant or his deputy. The trainee should prepare for this by having all case records (including previous volumes), drug prescription sheets, charts and investigation results to hand. Either the junior or senior trainee should discuss with the senior nurse the order in which the patients will be seen, taking into account new admissions, difficult clinical problems and the attendance of people such as probation officers who may be involved with only one patient.

For new patients the trainee should have prepared either a formulation (see Chapter 9) or a resumé of the history and mental state (see Chapters 10 and 6). Their length will partly be determined by the complexity of the case and how familiar the patient is to the team, and partly by the constraints imposed by the length of the ward round and the number of other patients to be seen. For the other patients the trainee needs to give a brief account of what has happened since the last ward round or review, paying particular attention to changes in mental state, changes in treatment, physical condition and investigation results. It is useful to remind the consultant exactly what each patient's current medication comprises.

After hearing about patients from various members of the team the consultant will usually see the patient and, if he is new to the psychiatric services, it is advisable for the trainee to have explained to the patient that the ward round usually involves the patient being seen in a room full of doctors, nurses and other involved staff. The trainee should record in the case records what the staff say about the patient and what takes place in the interview with the patient. Particular care should be taken to record accurately symptoms or signs which the consultant regards as being of diagnostic significance, answers to questions related to suicide risk, answers to questions concerning attitudes towards compliance with treatment and answers to questions concerning attitudes, beliefs or experiences which may make the patient potentially harmful towards others. From the discussion which follows the patient's interview the trainee should record the views concerning diagnosis, aetiology and prognosis and list the decisions made concerning the further assessment, care and treatment of the patient ('treatment plan'). It is useful to record who is responsible for the various elements and, if it is not clear who is doing what, to seek clarification before the next patient is discussed.

ADMISSIONS

Sometimes the trainee will be asked to arrange a patient's admission, in which case it is important to know about the administrative procedure for admissions. Few psychiatric hospitals or units follow a formal waiting-list procedure and once the degree of urgency has been established it is usually the responsibility of the trainee, secretary or nurse to ensure that the patient is admitted. Arrangements vary and the trainee should familiarise himself with the local procedure in order to ensure that patients are not overlooked, admitted to a no longer empty bed or arrive on wards where no one knows anything about them.

On the day of admission the patient should have a psychiatric history recorded and physical and mental state examinations recorded. How detailed the history is will be determined by a variety of factors but there must be nothing incomplete about the physical (Chapter 7) and mental state (Chapter 6) examinations. A patient's family history may not change from one day to the next but his mood or blood pressure may do. At the same time, if possible, an account of the patient's history should be taken from the relative who accompanies the patient and the opportunity used to explain what is likely to happen to the patient. Relatives may have a number of questions which they want to put to the doctor (see below). When history taking and examinations are complete it may be appropriate to carry out or organize some investigations (Chapter 8) and details of these should form part of the treatment plan recorded in the case records and discussed there and then with those staff, initially nurses, who are going to be involved in its implementation. It should be an explicit plan which makes quite clear what is to be done and by whom. It may include references to drug treatment prescribed (Chapters 12 and 13) and measures to be taken to provide appropriate care for a patient who is, for example, confused, over-active or potentially suicidal. Particularly in the case of patients whose diagnosis is as yet uncertain the trainee is likely to be taught to avoid the premature prescription of psychotropic drugs but some patients, particularly those needing treatment for physical illness, may have existing treatments continued. Subject to modification the treatment plan should provide the basis for organizing the patient's assessment and care until the next ward round or team meeting.

If the admission has not occurred with the knowledge of the general practitioner, he should be informed as soon as possible.

DISCHARGE

Patients' treatment rarely ceases when they leave hospital and whether or not their subsequent treatment is entirely in accord with the hospital team's expectations often depends upon the care with which the trainee coordinates discharge arrangements.

Family members need to know when a patient is to be expected or collected. Particularly if the patient will require fairly early attention from the primary health care team, it may be appropriate to discuss the patient's discharge with the general practitioner *before* it takes place. Appropriate arrangements may need to be made for the patient to be seen in the out-patient clinic.

A limited supply of drugs to be taken between discharge and the resumption of prescribing by the general practitioner may have to be organized and it is wise to check that all the drugs are actually required. The regime for taking the medication should be discussed with the patient and sometimes the relatives. Then they have the opportunity to ask again what the drugs are for and what effects they may have. Patients who have been started on a depot antipsychotic drug may need to have an appointment made for a special depot clinic.

A discharge letter to the general practitioner, sometimes with a copy to other involved specialists, needs to be prepared. Most psychiatric hospitals and units have a pre-printed standardized 'Preliminary Discharge Letter' which is completed on discharge and either posted by first-class mail to the general practitioner or placed in a sealed envelope for the patient or relative to give to the general practitioner at the earliest opportunity. Some patients cannot be trusted with such a letter and some consultants insist that all such letters are sent by post. It is important that the trainee ascertains the views of his own consultant. A carbon copy of the letter is usually filed in the case records. As soon as possible after discharge a full discharge summary should be prepared. Some consultants send general practitioners a copy of the discharge summary (Chapter 10), while others send general practitioners a discharge letter. Again the trainee needs to find out what practice his consultant prefers and what information he is expected to put in the discharge letter.

The patient's discharge from hospital completes an episode in his psychiatric history and for statistical and epidemiological purposes the DHSS requires that such an episode should, if appropriate, be labelled with one or more diagnoses which can be coded according to the International Classification of Diseases and Causes of Death (ICD-9). (Some hospitals provide trainees with their own copies of its glossary of mental disorders.) Such diagnoses are recorded on the form HMR 1 at the front of the case records and it is often the responsibility of the junior trainee to provide these diagnoses. Care should be taken to ensure that they accurately reflect the team's views and, although the ICD does not contain operational definitions, diagnoses are applied as consistently as possible. This will be particularly important when managers apply 'performance indicators' to various psychiatric diagnoses.

OUTPATIENTS

Junior trainees will usually be involved in seeing new referrals and follow-up patients in the out-patient setting. At the beginning it is important to distinguish, if possible, between patients being referred for psychiatric management and patients about whom the general practitioner wants an opinion or advice. However, in their approach to the assessment of new referrals they will usually be guided by their consultant and present the patient to the consultant or sometimes their senior registrar who will complete the formulation of the patient and communicate with the general practitioner or other referring agent. In the event of the trainee having to write a letter to the general practitioner concerning a new patient or, as part of his training, draft a letter which eventually goes in the consultant's name, it may be worth noting the conclusions of studies of letters from psychiatrists to general practitioners. There is general satisfaction with rather full one to two page A4 typed letters, but the length of the letter reflects a compromise between providing a permanent, legible record of the details of the case and avoiding telling the general practitioner what he already knows.

In general these can be divided into three sections: the first covering reasons for referral and the diagnostic formulation with reference to relevant aspects of the history and mental state; the second covering aspects of family, personal and medical history, perhaps in the form of an aetiological formulation, and the third dealing with treatment plans and prognosis. The middle section, often dealing with information well-known to the general practitioner, is best kept as brief as possible, while the first and last sections can be expanded to ensure that the general practitioner's specific questions are answered, and it is made clear how the patient is to be treated, what the prognosis is, what the responsibility of the general practitioner is and, if appropriate, what the patient and relatives have been told and how they have reacted. Most general practitioners want more explanation – for example about how diagnoses have been reached, what the condition is, or why a particular treatment has been recommended.

Follow-up patients will not necessarily be seen by the consultant at each visit but the trainee should not hesitate to ask his consultant to see a follow-up patient and discuss the patient with him. It is for this reason that the junior trainee should not usually see patients if neither the consultant nor senior registrar is available for consultation during the course of the clinic. Follow-up patients should not usually be discharged from a clinic by a junior trainee without this being discussed with the consultant. When writing letters concerning follow-up patients it is important to document, with the greatest possible brevity and clarity, details of significant recent events, recommendations for changes in medication (dose, dosage schedule, duration of administration etc.), other changes in treatment and what is expected of the general practitioner in the meantime. Letters to general practitioners should be sent as soon as possible after the patient has been seen and, if another specialist is also involved, particularly if he is likely to make his own recommendations concerning medication, it is important to send a copy of the letter to him. All letters sent by trainees should incorporate the name of the responsible consultant.

Except in emergencies outpatients should not be referred directly to other specialists. The general practitioner should be advised of the need for referral and allowed to refer the patient to a consultant of his choice.

DAY PATIENTS

Some patients may attend a day hospital and others may attend the ward or in-patient unit on a day patient basis. For some, but not all, assessment and treatment often takes place at a slower pace than that of in-patients and the trainee may not see them so frequently as in-patients. However, they require the same diligence in history taking, the documentation of psychopathology, monitoring of medication effects and side-effects and communication with others involved in their care. Day hospitals vary in their policies concerning prescribing, so it is important to ensure that both hospital doctor and general practitioner know who is prescribing what.

TALKING TO RELATIVES

Particularly when a patient has been newly admitted or is first seen in the out-patient clinic, it is easy for the busy trainee to regard a relative as little more than a source of information concerning the patient's mental state and history. However, relatives have their needs, and as well as meeting the needs of another, sometimes more distressed, person, an empathic and understanding response to the relative or relatives can prepare the way for the establishment of a positive approach to the patient, which could make all the difference to his treatment and rehabilitation. Such a response may call for an understanding of the relative which is as full as that of the patient and although such an understanding may not be present at the outset, it is a reasonable goal, particularly when family factors are important in the aetiology, treatment response and course of the patient's disorder.

For some relatives psychiatric referral or admission provides the opportunity to finally confide in someone what an awful time they have had for weeks, months or even years. For others it raises worrying questions about their own sanity or that of their children. For some it brings into sharp focus feelings of guilt concerning their own role in the patient's breakdown, guilt concerning the failure of family and other support systems to prevent the patient's referral or admission. For patients such as acute psychotics and parasuicide patients, admitted with relatively little warning, there may be anger about the involvement of the psychiatric services and more so where family, community, cultural, or architectural factors have perpetuated the stigma of psychiatric disorder. There may be a mixture, indeed an uncomfortable mixture, of feelings when, for example, a spouse or partner, already decided upon separation, finds herself overwhelmed by a sense of loyalty towards and responsibility for a partner whose acute illness is going to give way to chronic distress and dependency. The trainee must be sensitive to such feelings and encourage their expression.

Relatives will often want to know what is wrong, what the treatment is, how long it will take and what the outcome will be. Often it may be difficult to answer these questions when they are first asked. Rather than explain diagnoses which turn out to be wrong, make reassurances which do not stand the test of time or predictions which turn out to be incorrect, the trainee might initially be honest about the diagnostic, therapeutic or prognostic uncertainty and restrict reassurance to an account of the care which will be taken in assessment and diagnosis and the concern, understanding and skill of those who will be involved in the patient's care. Where the trainee's consultant or any other member of the team has particular expertise with the sort of problem presented by the patient this should be mentioned.

When it comes to explaining diagnoses, treatment and prognoses to relatives, something which will usually take place after the patient has been assessed by the complete psychiatric team, the trainee needs to be able to explain in lay language the most common psychiatric syndromes or diagnoses such as schizophrenia, dementia and psychosis and also the most common psychiatric treatments or approaches to treatment such as supportive psychotherapy, antipsychotic drugs, systematic desensitization and ECT. The trainee needs also to be aware of popular misconceptions which may confuse patients or relatives such as schizophrenia being a 'Jekyll and Hyde' phenomenon and ECT being a behavioural treatment employing a punishment principle. The degree of simplification employed in explaining diagnosis or treatment will be determined by the recipient's degree of intellectual or psychological sophistication and the trainee may need to adjust the level according to the recipient's response. Although there is an increasing number of leaflets and books concerning psychiatric disorders and their treatment directed at lay readership and, with selection according to the nature of the educational aid and its proposed recipient, these may sometimes be used to augment what the trainee tells the relative, they are no substitute for dialogue. Their existence should not encourage the trainee to merely send relatives away to read a booklet.

The relationship between a patient and his relatives is not static and the trainee must be prepared to see relatives at intervals during the patient's treatment, responding where appropriate to their changing needs and feelings as well as responding to their desire for more information, different information or even the same information again.

Further reading

Carstairs GM, Early DF, Rollin HR and Wing JK (1985) Informing relatives about schizophrenia. *Bulletin of the Royal College of Psychiatrists 9:* 59–60

Margo JL (1982) Letters from psychiatrists to general practitioners. *Bulletin of the Royal College of Psychiatrists 6:* 139–141

National Schizophrenia Fellowship (1983) *Good Relations. A Code of Practice for those Discharging Patients.* Surbitan: NSF

Pullen IM and Yellowlees AJ (1985) Is communication improving between general practitioners and psychiatrists? *British Medical Journal 290:* 31–33

World Health Organisation (1978) *Mental Disorders: Glossary and Guide to their Classification in Accordance with the Ninth Revision of the International Classification of Diseases.* Geneva: WHO

— 3 —

Working with Fellow Professionals

J. P. Wattis

One of the great interests of psychiatry is that it involves the whole person. Biochemical and genetic factors are important in many of the more severe psychiatric disorders but even in these illnesses psychological, social, cultural and family factors can play a major part. Brown and his colleagues' work on the social factors in depression and Vaughan and others' work on the importance of family emotion in predicting schizophrenic relapse are good examples of this.

When patients are acutely ill, they may need nursing care to compensate for deficiencies in self care, to protect them from self-destructive behaviour or to protect others from inappropriate action. Nursing care is also directed to enable the person to return to independent living. Specific help may also be required from clinical psychologists, social workers, occupational therapists, physiotherapists, speech therapists and others. The management of mental disorder demands cooperation between members of different professions. The epitome of such cooperation is the properly functioning multi-disciplinary team. Often, however, there are rivalries and obstacles to multi-disciplinary working. Some have even asserted that multi-disciplinary teams erode medical responsibility and produce procrastination. This need not be so, but some of the reasons for difficulty in multi-disciplinary working will now be discussed.

PROFESSIONAL HISTORY

The medical profession, together with the priesthood and legal profession, has a long history. It has evolved a structure where the most senior posts are occupied by people still practising the profession, the consultant grade. Further, most teaching of the profession is in the hands of clinical practitioners. The medical profession has a strong knowledge base and is seen as meeting a real and important need in society. It has a long period of education with highly developed specialization and a strong tradition of professional autonomy even when, as in the NHS, the doctors are salaried employees. People going into medical training generally have to be very highly committed and tend to maintain that commitment through life. Medicine has a strong professional identity and its ethics have been identified since the time of Hippocrates. It has a fine tradition of altruistic service, although some would say this is being undermined by profit-seeking and an 'industrialization' of attitudes.

By contrast, the nursing profession is relatively young, has a less-developed knowledge base, tends to be taught and administered by those who are no longer practitioners and has less commitment (as measured by drop-out during and after training), and less professional autonomy than medicine. All the other professions with which doctors have to deal are also relatively young and emergent and it is all too easy for doctors to develop a superior attitude which is resented by other disciplines which perceive themselves as being regarded as inferior.

MEDICAL TRAINING

Perhaps because medicine is an ancient profession, training is slow to adapt to current realities. Many schools still teach anatomy, physiology and basic sciences to their pre-clinical students with little time for behavioural sciences, management skills or practical training in how to work with other disciplines. Doctors may therefore feel insecure in their relationships with other professions and react by adding arrogance to pride! More often than not the problem inflicted by the different stages of development of the professions, by differences and inadequacies in training and by other administrative problems to be discussed later, are overcome in the interests of working together for the sake of the patient. For the doctor and for other professionals this altruistic concern for the good of the patient must be the principle by which interdisciplinary relationships are governed.

RESPECT

Status

People who feel insecure often enhance their self-respect by denigrating others. They never earn the respect of others by this method! Junior doctors are often part of training rotations that only allow them to stay in one place for six months at a time. Although there are important advantages in such a scheme there are also major disadvantages. One of these, in the present context, is that they do not always have time to get to know professionals of other disciplines personally. In this kind of situation prejudices flourish. Some doctors have stereotypes of nurses as unintelligent. Some nurses see doctors as uncaring. Doctors may regard social workers as woolly-minded and irresponsible, whilst social workers may think that doctors are authoritarian and only capable of treating people with drugs and electroconvulsive therapy. Of course any of these statements might be true about some doctors, some nurses or some social workers some of the time, but to believe that they apply universally is an insult to the individuality of people working in these disciplines. The aphorism "He who generalizes, generally lies" is highly appropriate here.

The antidote to stereotyping is getting to know other people in other disciplines more closely, recognizing that the medical profession does not have a monopoly on effective treatment for mental disorder and striving to understand the values and motives of one's colleagues in other professions. Sometimes people complain that multi-disciplinary team meetings are too 'chatty' and wander too far from discussion of particular patients and sometimes, of course, they are right. On the other hand, often such free-ranging discussions are a vehicle of education for all the disciplines involved.

Ethics and values

Each discipline has its own ethics and values. Medical ethics have a very long history and other professions have often borrowed some of the principles of medical ethics. Nevertheless, there can sometimes be a clash because of the different importance attached to different judgments and issues by different professionals. The doctor is firmly trained in a scientific way of thinking. He is taught to elicit evidence from the history and mental state of the patient on which to base a diagnosis which has definite implications for treatment and prognosis. Working within this framework of relative certainty the doctor in England and Wales may confidently believe that it is essential for the patient to be admitted or treated, even if compulsory powers under the Mental Health Act (1983) have to be invoked. Coming from a different background, the social worker, with a greater relative emphasis on the value of freedom for the individual (even if to the doctor that merely seems freedom to be unnecessarily ill), and less certainty about the outcome of treatment, may be unwilling to make the necessary application.* The junior doctor will not usually be directly involved in such a drama, but may stand in the wings as consultant and social worker strive for a resolution. There are several possible outcomes. The consultant who is sufficiently respected may be able to demonstrate to the social worker's satisfaction that an

---

*In Scotland such disputes are less likely since the arrangements for compulsory admission are different – see p.210

application is necessary. The social worker who is sufficiently respected may be able to show the consultant that there are proper alternatives to compulsory admission or treatment. The consultant may seek by one means or another to override the social worker; indeed the consultant may feel ethically obliged to do so. In this kind of situation a satisfactory solution is usually only achieved if both protagonists respect each other and are prepared to concede that the other person's solution, while not ideal, might be feasible. A combination of concern for what is best for the patient and determination to avoid a simple power-struggle is essential.

UNDERSTANDING AND COMMUNICATION

Respect and understanding are closely linked. If we respect people we will usually take the trouble to understand their point of view. We must also try to understand the extent and the limits of training in other disciplines. When asked one thing he would like to communicate to junior doctors through this chapter, a very experienced and capable social welfare officer said that he wanted to be treated as "ignorant". By this he meant that doctors should not assume that he understood the rationale behind a particular medical treatment, but that they should explain this to him. He, in turn, would be willing to explain facets of his job to the junior trainee.

Overlapping functions

Figure 3.1 is a diagram to illustrate overlapping functions. For simplicity it is limited to three disciplines, though in reality many more disciplines may be involved. The central area ('A' in the diagram) represents shared skills. For example, it is quite feasible, though not necessary, that social workers, psychiatric nurses and doctors might share skills in bereavement counselling. Area B represents skills that are not shared

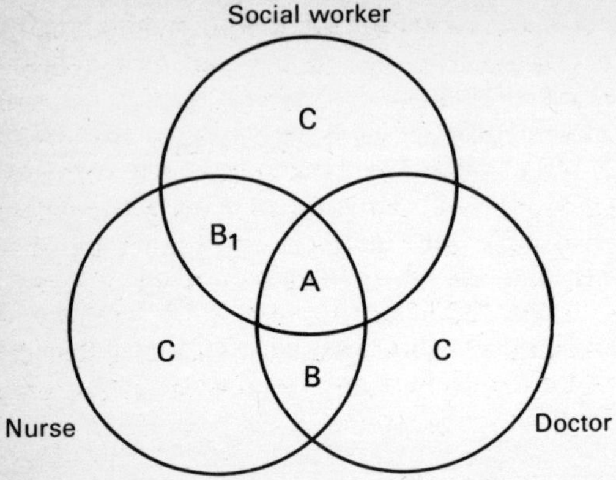

Fig. 3.1 Overlapping functions in the multidisciplinary team. (Reproduced with thanks and minor modifications from Wattis J and Church M (1986) *Practical Psychiatry of Old Age.* London: Croom Helm.)

by all disciplines, for example, doctors and nurses are both trained to give injections, social workers are not. Area C is the area of unique skill; perhaps medical diagnosis and treatment for the doctor, 24-hour nursing care and certain aspects of community care for the nurse, setting up social support networks and mediating between client and officialdom for the social worker. To some extent these boundaries are flexible and vary according to the particular people concerned and their personal experience and training, to some extent they are fixed by law or custom.

There is sometimes a tendency for workers of all disciplines to migrate into the more 'attractive' central areas of working to the neglect of the rather tedious routine of their own specialized discipline's area. Leaders within the team have to detect and counter this. There is also a problem about recognizing other people's talents and training. Multi-disciplinary courses, in psychotherapy for example, can help overcome this. Sometimes one discipline may have a much more rigorous training in a particular area than another. Some clinical psychologists, for example, will be much better at putting together a behaviour modification programme than some doctors or nurses. As long as people are prepared to recognize and concede another's greater expertise this raises no problems. If a worker of whatever discipline believes that he or she has skills (for example in psychotherapy) that he or she patently has not, then there is a major problem. Great skills may be needed in other members of the team, perhaps of other disciplines, to safeguard the patient and at the same time tactfully point out the problem without 'putting down' the team member in question.

Structural problems

Amongst all the disciplines working in health care, medicine is unique in that responsibility rests fully on a clinically active person, the consultant. The team can be represented diagrammatically as a 'flattened pyramid' of authority with the consultant at the top (Figure 3.2). All the medical members of

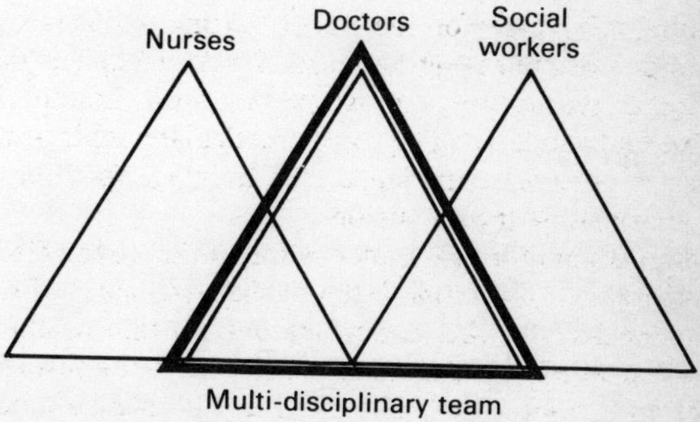

Fig. 3.2 Structure of the multi-disciplinary team. (Reproduced with thanks from Wattis J and Church M (1986) *Practical Psychiatry of Old Age.* London: Croom Helm.)

the team 'report to' the consultant who has overall responsibility for medical care. On the other hand the most senior clinical nurse or social worker within the team reports to a senior outside of the team, who usually is not involved in any kind of clinical work, let alone the work of the team. This difference in status (clearly represented by salary differentials) between the consultant and the most senior non-medical members of the team can pose major problems if not handled with sensitivity. If the nursing and social work higher management are prepared to delegate responsibility so that the senior professionals within the team are more or less autonomous, this will help. If not, major problems can arise when, for example, a nurse or social worker in the team is overridden by a more senior member of the same discipline. Other disciplines may be more subject to bureaucratic and even (in the case of social workers) local political control, than doctors. Even when workers are relatively autonomous their power to 'deliver' may vary depending on local circumstances. The doctor who, under the consultant, has absolute authority to admit a patient to an acute or long-stay bed, may find it hard to accept the fact that the social worker has to leave the decision about whether or not a patient/client should go into residential care to a committee who have never seen the subject of their deliberations.

Communication

Just as understanding and communication are at the heart of successful psychotherapy, so they are at the heart of successful team work. Referring a patient for help to a member of another discipline is best done by word of mouth as well as by printed form. Discussion about the aptness of the referral is then possible. At times a task in the shared area (B_1 in Figure 3.1) may be taken on by the community nurse because the social worker is too busy or vice versa. Physical proximity encourages communication and an open-plan multi-disciplinary office is a practical move towards encouraging team work.

A weekly referral meeting when all new referrals to the team (who may already have been assessed by a senior doctor) are briefly discussed in the presence of all disciplines, also helps establish good communication. In some cases the discussion will enable new suggestions for management to emerge. This kind of forum can also provide an opportunity for members of all disciplines to raise issues concerning ongoing patients for the advice and help of other professionals.

TEAM WORK AND LEADERSHIP

Team work is time-consuming. A consistent criticism by rotating junior doctors and others is the time spent in meetings. Unfortunately true team work is impossible without frequent meetings at a formal and informal level. Apart from the doctors, other disciplines in the team will belong to their own disciplinary team which extends beyond the 'flattened pyramid' of the multi-disciplinary team structure. If a multi-disciplinary team is to work properly, it is essential that this does not produce a conflict of loyalties. To achieve this the multi-disciplinary team needs sensitive leadership. For the structural reasons already noted, the consultant is probably the 'natural' leader for most multi-disciplinary teams. However, not all consultants have the necessary leadership skills. Fortunately these skills can be acquired and leadership training should be part of the training of every junior doctor. Leadership can be 'imposed' or come out of the common consent of all members of the team ('emergent' leadership). If the 'imposed' leader and the 'emergent' leader are not one and the same person there can be major problems. What then suits a person to become an 'emergent' leader? First the person must have the authority of a broad and secure knowledge base, second he must be strongly committed to a particular goal (e.g. providing psychiatric services for old people/the general adult population/children). Then he must be able to understand and respect the point of view of other disciplines and communicate that understanding and respect. There is a continuum of leadership from the totally authoritarian to the totally permissive. Most successful leaders operate somewhere in the middle of this continuum, in the style usually referred to as 'democratic' or (slightly more authoritarian) 'diplomatic'. The degree of permissiveness will also vary with the subject under discussion. If it is a question of a specific medical treatment the doctor may feel that he can be more prescriptive. If the issue is, for example, more in the social realm, he should generally defer to those with more expertise than himself.

The concept of a 'key worker' is particularly useful in community psychiatry. Here a worker, of whatever discipline, takes key responsibility for coordinating a patient's management and all new information and decisions are, as far as possible, channelled through him. This enables all members of the team to share the leadership role in particular cases. Team work does raise questions of confidentiality. Provided that the patient or his relatives understand that the approach being adopted is a team approach and provided all professions in the team agree to keep confidences within the team this should not be a problem.

In conclusion, team work is essential to modern psychiatry. Effective team work is in the best interests of the patient. It can only be achieved if different disciplines show mutual respect and understanding and if the leadership function imposed on the doctor by administrative and other constraints is matched by a leadership ability which causes other professions to concede the overall leadership role, whilst retaining for themselves the leadership role in particular situations and cases where circumstances make it appropriate.

Further reading

Appleyard J and Maden JG (1979) Multidisciplinary teams. *British Medical Journal 2:* 1305–1307

Bebbington PE and Hill PD (1985) Working with colleagues. In *A Manual of Practical Psychiatry*, pp.328–341. Oxford: Blackwell

Bernhard LA and Walsh M (1981) *Leadership: the Key to the Professionalization of Nursing.* New York: McGraw-Hill

Wattis JP (1979) Multidisciplinary teams (Letter). *British Medical Journal 2:* 1509

4

Working as Duty Psychiatrist

Francis Creed

DEMANDS ON THE SERVICE

Calls to the service come from many sources. Out of hours the duty psychiatrist may be contacted by general practitioners, other hospital doctors, the police, social workers, community nurses and probation officers. Some hospital switchboards put through calls from patients, ex-patients and relatives. The nature of these calls varies. Some are simply for advice, others request an assessment or admission. However much a call seems 'inappropriate' the trainee should try and be patient and understanding. He may be in a position to help a distressed relative or professional who is facing a problem with which they feel unable to cope. Although the behaviour of a psychotic or depressed patient may be familiar to the trainee, for the person on the other end of the line it may be the first experience and very frightening.

The duty psychiatrist will be expected to deal with most of the calls himself, but he should know beforehand which calls should be put through to a more senior psychiatrist.

The duty psychiatrist will be required to be available within the hospital for emergencies concerning in-patients, patients brought to the casualty department and emergency assessments requested by other doctors. He should be clear of the policy regarding the last of these. Some departments have a policy of only seeing patients referred by other doctors. Others see patients referred by themselves, relatives or social workers.

The office used to see such patients out of hours needs to be somewhere private enough for a proper consultation but within easy reach of several nurses who can immediately accompany the doctor if a disturbed or potentially violent patient is to be seen. It ought to have a 'panic button', fixed furniture which cannot be used in a violent outburst, a seat for the doctor which is within easy reach of the door and perhaps a 'spy-hole' in the door. There should be no heavy metal or glass ashtrays or other objects which might be used to attack the doctor.

As with assessments of patients from the community, those in the wards of the general hospital who require urgent assessment will fall to the duty doctor and routine referrals should be referred to a senior psychiatrist.

SUPERVISION OF THE DUTY PSYCHIATRIST

Although he may be quite junior, the duty psychiatrist inevitably represents the psychiatry service out of hours. For this reason it is preferable if a new trainee is closely supervised during his first few times on call or even not required to do a duty until he has been in the specialty for a month. It is usually the case that the duty psychiatrist has to work in relative isolation compared to the multi-disciplinary team available during the daytime or the fully staffed accident and emergency department.

This means that it is a challenging and difficult job which requires a close relationship between the duty doctor and the senior on call. It is helpful if the latter checks with the duty doctor about any current or potential problems before going home in the evening.

Contrary to popular belief, a common complaint from senior psychiatrists is that they are not consulted frequently enough by the duty doctor. This is because major problems of management can be created by an inappropriate admission but avoided if alternative management is found at the time of crisis.

BEFORE COMMENCING DUTY

The trainee should check who else is on call and when they expect to hear from him.

He must be clear about the times of duty. This may seem obvious, but attempts to contact the duty doctor around 5pm can lead to the conclusion that no-one is accepting responsibility for calls at that moment. This is frustrating and can occasionally lead to impulsive action by a busy referring doctor, such as sending a patient up to the hospital unannounced. The ensuing management difficulties are ones which should have been avoided.

It is important that the bleep be passed directly from one duty doctor to another and *not* left on a particular ward to be collected at a certain time. The latter practice fails because the doctor coming on call occasionally gets held up and this is the moment that a senior general practitioner rings! It is also essential that the doctor going off duty tells the new doctor what problems are pending. Once the bleep has been picked up, it should not be put down unless there is someone who can be reliably trusted to disturb the duty doctor if he is needed urgently. A quick word immediately can save a lot of trouble later.

This message cannot be over-emphasized. Consider the senior registrar or consultant who has just done an urgent domiciliary visit, organized a compulsory admission and used his last ten pence piece to inform the duty doctor of the relevant clinical details. "Can you ring back in five minutes because the duty doctor is with a patient at present?" sounds a bit hollow then!

THE DUTY BOOK(S)

In a well-run service there will be two books for the duty psychiatrist. One concerns general procedures that the duty psychiatrist is expected to follow. The other is a book that contains details of on-going problems to which the doctor may be called. Examples of such problems include a self-poisoning patient too drowsy to be assessed previously, or a patient about whom a policy decision has already been made regarding admission or prescription. This book should be a continuing source of active problems so the duty doctor is as likely to contribute to it as derive information from it. Should neither book exist the divisional chairman should be told that they are needed. Some hospitals combine these books in the form of a single loose-leaf book which can be constantly updated.

The book or books should contain certain basic information:

- A map or other means of determining if an address is inside the catchment area.
- The relevant hospitals for patients living in neighbouring areas (senior nursing staff are usually invaluable sources of such information, including which doctor should be approached in each hospital – some duty doctors in residence deal with admissions; others require the involvement of the duty consultant from the outset).
- Useful telephone numbers including:
  –Neighbouring hospitals
  –Local poisoning service
  –Local Authority social services emergency number
  –Telephone number of any specialist teams that are available out of hours, such as psychogeriatrician, mental handicap team, community nurses or crisis team.

There should also be guidelines for certain circumstances and procedures:

- Arrangements for *patients over 65 years* who sound as though they may be dementing. Is it a problem with which the duty doctor becomes involved or is the referral put straight through to a psychogeriatrician who only admits following a domiciliary visit?
- Arrangements for *emergency assessments* of patients out of hours at the hospital, at a police station, or at home.

- Under which consultant a patient is admitted. This depends on local policy – by address, by previous care or by firm on take. The duty doctor must be familiar with the admission procedure, know where the vacant beds are or be clear where he can gain this knowledge.
- How to obtain *records* out of hours.
- The arrangements for *compulsory admissions*, e.g. what happens if a general practitioner insists on admitting a patient under Section 4? (see Chapter 16).
- Who signs *Section 5(2)* (see Chapter 16).
- When and where the duty doctor gets his *supper*.
- The range of the *bleep*.
- The arrangement for getting *emergency drugs* from the pharmacy.

FORMS AND FILES

All transactions involving patients must be recorded by the duty doctor in the duty book and/or in the patient's notes (see p.16).

If there are no psychiatric records, any dealings with or about a patient should be recorded in the duty book and the clinical details must be recorded on the referral sheet from the physician or surgeon. For example, there may be telephone calls with other hospitals and the general practitioner about a difficult self-poisoning patient who is still drowsy. The information thus gained must be recorded for subsequent duty doctors.

For a patient admitted to the psychiatric ward the exact circumstances leading up to admission must be clearly recorded in the case records in addition to the usual history and mental state. If a loose-leaf duty book is used it can hold a small number of forms which may be required during the course of duty: Drug Addiction Notification forms, ward referral forms, most relevant Mental Health Act forms, case history and examination sheets.

Many hospitals have a special consultation sheet, the first half of which is completed by the referring doctor and the second half by the duty psychiatrist. (If the referral is addressed to a named consultant, the trainee must ensure that the case is discussed with him.) This sheet should *always* be completed by both parties. It is preferable for the duty doctor not to see the patient without such a form, so that it is clear who is responsible for the patient and why the referral is being requested.

SPECIFIC PROBLEMS

The duty psychiatrist can find himself under pressure to decide and act quickly with a complex clinical situation that even a more senior person would require time and thought to sort out properly. For example, a general practitioner may request urgent admission for a confused elderly patient or the casualty staff may be pressing for the compulsory admission of a potentially violent or apparently suicidal patient, when positive evidence for mental illness is lacking.

In such situations it is often difficult to obtain the history from an informant which is required for a full assessment. Without it one is making a decision on the mental state alone. This is occasionally necessary (and corresponds to the care of the unconscious patient in general medicine), but is open to all sorts of hazards. The assessment of an apparently suicidal person can change dramatically when the psychiatrist discovers that the patient was discharged from a psychiatric hospital the previous day, having been diagnosed as a sociopathic personality whose persistent hospitalizations were considered to be counterproductive in the long term.

Call from general practitioner about a possible admission

It is annoying and unnecessary for a general practitioner to relay the details of a patient twice, so the duty doctor should politely ascertain early in the conversation whether the patient can be brought to the hospital for assessment, or a home visit is being requested. In the latter case, it may be preferable for the general practitioner to speak directly to the senior on call who will do the visit.

The decision to bring a patient to the hospital may be a far-reaching one. It usually raises the expectations of admission both in the mind of the patient or of his attendants. This may not be helpful. For a patient seeking admission it makes refusal more difficult. For the relatives it may imply that the effort to maintain the patient at home is over. In the case of the police it may indicate that the psychiatry service is assuming responsibility for a (usually disturbed) patient when the psychiatrist's role is to examine the patient for evidence of mental illness (see p.220). There may be occasions when the duty doctor is unsure whether to arrange for the patient to come to the hospital so a discussion with the senior on call is needed first. When the patient is to come to the hospital it is advisable to point out that the purpose of the visit is to assess the patient's mental state, so admission is not in any way guaranteed. It is important that relatives or other carers accompany the patient.

At the hospital, the duty doctor and attendant nurses should try and be aware of the anxieties and expectations of the patient and his accompanying relatives. More than the usual care is needed to manage the assessment interview, even if the patient is not apparently disturbed. Many patients attending the routine out-patient clinic have unreasonable fears about what is going to happen to them; these fears will be heightened at a time of crisis.

It is usually convenient for the psychiatrist to get an objective history from an informant first, and then assess the patient's mental state. This may be asking too much of some patients, who may become suspicious or irritable while waiting. So it is usually best for the doctor to speak briefly to the patient first in order to gain his confidence and an outline of the problem. Then he should speak with the relatives, ensuring that someone (preferably a nurse) is supervising the patient. Finally the doctor should speak again to the patient, clarifying the details of the account given by the relatives, and assess the mental state.

Difficulties arise when the relative reports that a patient has been disturbed in his behaviour, but the patient denies such behaviour and appears calm at interview. In this situation the doctor must be sure of his facts before putting them to the patient. These will be gained firstly by a clear account over the telephone prior to the assessment, and secondly, during the interview with the relative without the patient present.

The management plan should be explained clearly to both parties once the doctor has decided what to do.

The possible lines of action are:

- immediate admission either to the in-patient unit or the day hospital,
- an urgent out-patient appointment either with the duty doctor himself or another doctor,
- a routine appointment with the appropriate psychiatrist or referral to another agency (e.g. psychologist, specialist team, social worker),
- referral back to the general practitioner.

The duty doctor must clearly state who is continuing to be responsible for the patient. He should preferably speak with the responsible doctor, or other professional, either immediately or the next working day. It is only once this contact by phone and/or letter has been accomplished that the duty doctor's task has been completed. Too often there is inadequate effort expended with this last task which may leave the patient and his relatives no better off than prior to the assessment. The duty doctor should do his best to ensure that an urgent appointment is made if that is the outcome of his assessment.

It should become routine that the duty doctor completes letters or telephone calls first thing on the next working day before he becomes involved in his routine work.

Call to attend an in-patient

The principles are similar whether the patient is in a general or a psychiatric ward. The duty doctor should follow these steps:

1. He should establish on the telephone from the referring doctor (or nurse if a psychiatric ward) the exact nature of the request. He can then decide whether to attend immediately or finish his present task first.

2. He must be prepared to speak at some length to the nurse on the ward about the nature of the present crisis. There may have been a similar episode before and it is appropriate to ask what the response was previously. The duty doctor should ask if a contingency plan has already been established at a ward round. He will also establish something of the background of the patient's illness and line of treatment from the nurse.

He must be clear exactly why he is seeing the patient. The aim of the interview may be to elicit information, or it might be to enforce a line of management. If the doctor is asked to see a patient who is threatening to discharge himself the first task is to assess suicidal risk, the second task is to make a decision and the third is to discuss or enforce the management plan. Only an experienced psychiatrist can do all three simultaneously; the trainee is best advised to keep the tasks separate initially, especially as he may need to discuss the decision with the senior on call.

3. The doctor should carefully read the records, firstly to establish the diagnosis and plan of treatment, and secondly to see if any instructions have been left in the event of a crisis; there may be clear instructions to consider compulsory detention if the patient intends to leave or to consider discharge if he is too disruptive or exceeds specific limits.

It may become clear that a senior member of the responsible team should be contacted, especially if the trainee feels it is inappropriate to follow the instructions in the notes because the patient's clinical state has changed. An example would be the alcohol-dependent patient who has broken his contract by drinking, but who seems now to be a clear suicidal risk. Similarly the severely depressed patient who has become stuporose might best be managed by arranging ECT on the following day, but this requires discussion with the responsible team.

The duty doctor should check in the notes for known allergies to certain drugs that he might consider using.

4. Only after these preliminary steps should the doctor see the patient. The more information he has gained before seeing the patient the better the interview will be. A very tense patient will not describe her worries clearly to a stranger, but will speak more freely to the doctor who is obviously aware of her concerns (e.g. the anniversary of her mother's death, her preoccupation about the children or the effects of her medication).

5. The doctor must decide what action to take; this usually requires discussion with the nursing staff and possibly discussion with the senior on call also.

6. The doctor must ensure that the nursing staff are clear what has been decided and why, making sure that they can implement the management plan – e.g. that they have enough nurses to detain the patient if necessary. Any medication that is prescribed (either by the duty doctor, or the houseman on a general medical ward), must be immediately available and the duty doctor should be present while it is administered if the patient is potentially violent. If the patient is physically ill and cannot tolerate sedation, the nurses on the general ward will need counselling as how best to manage the patient. It is often helpful for a nurse from the psychiatric ward to go over to the medical ward for this purpose. The trainee should not underestimate the importance of discussing the management problem with the nursing staff. If they are having to cope with a disturbed and uncooperative patient, listening carefully to their complaints and promising to emphasize these to the regular doctors can often enable them to continue being tolerant of a difficult nursing situation.

7. The doctor should document in the patient's records the nature of the crisis, the mental state, the names of the doctors with whom the problem was discussed and what management was taken. He should ensure that the nursing staff will contact the patient's regular doctor at the first opportunity and anything relevant should be recorded in the duty book.

Assessment of the parasuicide patient

This assessment should be done under the usual headings. In the history there are four main areas:

- Detailed history of the circumstances of the parasuicide.
  (a) Objective – degree of isolation, timing and precautions to avoid discovery, suicide note or other act in anticipation of death; any relevant action after the act.
  (b) Subjective – stated intent, patient's estimate of lethality of dose taken, premeditation.
- Any evidence of recent/current psychiatric illness, especially depressive or psychotic illness.
- Any history of previous parasuicide, or psychiatric illness in the patient or his family.
- Evidence of alcohol and drug abuse are sought.

The mental state is assessed as usual, but evidence of depressed mood and continuing suicidal ideation is particularly relevant. Psychotic phenomena, attitude towards the parasuicide and continuing treatment may also determine immediate management. For many parasuicide patients this assessment leads to a clear management plan. There may be no continuing risk of further self-harm and the patient may be discharged or this risk may be considerable, in which case admission to the psychiatric unit is advisable. Management is less clear in the following circumstances:

– when the risk of further self-harm appears slight, but the psychiatrist feels uneasy about letting the patient go home,
– when the patient is determined to go home immediately even though the psychiatrist feels there is some risk of further self-harm, and

– if the patient has a long history of repeated parasuicide and there is a general feeling that admission to the psychiatric unit is unhelpful in the long term.

With these difficult problems the trainee should consider consulting the senior on call. This may be to:

– clarify his thoughts about the case and gain advice regarding further action (for example, a satisfactory decision may be impossible without further information e.g. from another hospital, or the warden of the hostel where the patient lives),

– to discuss with another psychiatrist the 'pros' and 'cons' of admission (i.e. reduce the isolation of the duty psychiatrist),

– shift responsibility to a more senior person (which is the reason for having a senior person on call, so the trainee must not be shy about this),

– to learn more about this type of problem and its management. Too often emergency work falls outside the scope of routine clinical supervision, which is a mistake because there is much to learn from an experienced psychiatrist regarding emergency work,

– to clarify whether a patient is sufficiently 'physically fit' to be discharged or transferred to the psychiatric unit. This decision often appears to be made by others, but the patient who shows mild clouding of consciousness undetected by the referring doctor may not be ready for transfer or discharge.

Any one of these reasons may lead to the senior psychiatrist coming to see the patient himself. The duty doctor should try and make it clear that he finds the assessment difficult, in which case it is appropriate for the senior to see the patient, or whether he is uncertain about the correct management when in full possession of all the facts. The latter can more often be dealt with over the telephone.

The drug-dependent patient

Drug-dependent patients can cause enormous problems to the duty doctor. They should not. A proper procedure for patients attending the casualty department requesting drugs, begins with clear instructions to the casualty staff as to the hospital's policy. Such a policy is laid down by the relevant divisions and clearly written down. It is not decided by duty staff.

If there is no prescription of methadone or equivalent drug other than at a drug-dependence clinic the casualty staff can convey this to patients without the psychiatrist being involved. Relaying such an official policy is easier than justifying an individual decision not to prescribe. Duty doctors must realise that relevant information may be widely disseminated among drug users. If one patient does manage to gain a prescription for opiates or any psychotropic drug at a casualty department, this may be followed by many more such requests. But if a firm no-prescription policy is always followed, such requests will become very rare.

If the duty psychiatrist does see a drug-dependent patient he should consider whether or not there is a statutory obligation to notify the Home Office Drugs Branch (see BNF for details).

CONCLUDING REMARKS

Finally, the duty psychiatrist should try and plan his work. There are times when this seems impossible because of the many demands that occur simultaneously, but he should be aware of the relative urgency of each request, and if possible deal with each one as it appears. The division of psychiatry should arrange that routine requests for assessment of self-poisoning patients reach the department early in the morning. This enables the duty doctor to deal with them while the daytime staff (social workers and other psychiatry units) are available. The ward staff can also be asked to arrange for a relative to be on the ward when the duty doctor is going to assess the patient.

Clear notes, both in the patient's file and in the duty books, are essential – these notes should be made as the doctor deals with problems. Returning to this task at a later time is inefficient and leads to omissions.

Trainees occasionally require reminding of medico-legal implications, such as recording suicidal status for depressed patients. They should always try to avoid being alone with a potentially violent patient. Keeping in touch with the senior on call is important: he or she is there to help the trainee and not judge him, and will probably have experienced a situation similar himself. Emergency psychiatry is not dull and there is much to be learned!

Further reading

Bowker M and McGrath G (1986) *Common Psychiatric Emergencies.* Bristol: John Wright

Waldron G (1982) Psychiatric emergencies. In Creed F and Pfeffer J, eds. *Medicine and Psychiatry – A Practical Approach,* pp.86–104. London: Pitman Medical

5

Interviewing Skills

Peter Maguire

As a psychiatrist you need to interview in a way which encourages patients to trust you and fully and honestly disclose all relevant information. Otherwise your diagnosis and plan of management will be based on inadequate data. You also have to establish patients' views about their illness, possible causes and treatments, for these must be taken into account if you are to persuade them to accept and comply with your treatment and advice. Ways of achieving these goals will be discussed.

THE SETTING

Whenever possible you should see patients in private and avoid interruptions. This is most difficult to achieve when you assess patients on general medical and surgical wards or in casualty. However, it is important that you are tough-minded about this, since this will demonstrate your concern for your patients' welfare and your determination to avoid their personal problems becoming public knowledge. Unless privacy is achieved, patients may hold back important information because they believe they might be overheard by fellow patients or members of staff.

Having established privacy it is important to arrange the seating so that there is no physical barrier between you and the patient such as a desk. It is also useful to avoid sitting face-to-face. Otherwise, eye contact will be experienced as discomforting rather than helpful. Chairs set at right angles or a slightly greater angle are optimal.

This chapter can be read alongside Chapter 10, which details the areas of information covered in psychiatric interviews.

THE BEGINNING

When meeting a patient for the first time you should introduce yourself and explain your status, for example, "I'm Clare Williams, a registrar in psychiatry working for Dr Jones", since patients often do not realise who has assessed them and may not have been told that they are seeing a psychiatrist. The patient should then be shown the chair he/she is to sit on and given a moment to sit down and settle before you begin the interview.

ORIENTATION

Most patients who are seeing a psychiatrist for the first time do not know what to expect. So, you should begin by explaining that you would like to focus on their presenting problems, that is, the changes that have occurred recently which have led them to be referred to you. This will minimize the possibility that you will fall into a common trap. When psychiatric patients are asked what brought them to hospital, they commonly launch into an explanation of why they think they have become ill. This can result in lengthy accounts of how a marriage has broken down or how other chronic difficulties developed, like housing or financial problems. The interviewer will then learn more about possible aetiological factors than the nature and severity of the clinical problems. Making the goals of the interview explicit from the outset will also allow you to exert control if the patient gets off the point, for you can remind the patient gently that the prime focus should be on his or her presenting problem.

You should next mention the time you have available, for example "We have up to 45 minutes today if we need it". This is usually acceptable, since it represents a much longer time than patients expect when they visit a doctor – for example, when they visit their general practitioner they expect 5 to 10 minutes. Having explained the focus of the interview and the time available, you should negotiate this with your patient by enquiring "Is that all right?". The patient can then indicate that he/she would prefer the interview to proceed in some other way, or that the time available is too much ("There's no way I'll need that amount of time") or too little ("I'm afraid I've so much to tell you that I don't think I can possibly do it justice in that time"). If the latter response occurs you can indicate "Well, in that case I'll arrange to see you for a further interview very soon, but let's see how far we can get today; all right?".

NOTE-TAKING

You should then explain that you would like to take notes to help you remember what you have discussed and negotiate this ("I'd like to take some notes to help me remember what we've talked about; is that all right?"). Most patients will agree, but some may voice disquiet or show this non-verbally. When they do so, you should explore their reasons fully and respect them if they are salient, for example "I'm not sure I can trust you; I keep worrying that you're a member of the KGB as well; I'd rather you didn't take notes", or "I don't mind you taking notes as long as when I get to the problems with my wife, you leave them out".

Some psychiatrists argue that note-taking prevents you establishing an effective relationship, and they prefer that you do not take any notes. But you are then likely to forget important data. Moreover, patients will regard your note-taking as a sign that you are interested in them, particularly if what you note down reflects their view of what is important, and you maintain reasonable eye contact by ensuring that you look up at the end of each utterance. If the patient gives any verbal or non-verbal signals during this orientation phase that he/she is unhappy or distressed by what is proposed, it is important that you acknowledge this and explore the reasons. Some patients are not warned that they are seeing a psychiatrist or realise this and fear they will be judged mad, kept in hospital against their will and given hazardous treatments like ECT or strong sedatives.

Doctor You don't seem very happy about what I'm proposing?
Patient I'm not.
Doctor Would you mind telling me why?
Patient No I wouldn't. I didn't want to come and see you in the first place. It's bad enough having cancer but to have to come and see a psychiatrist as well is the last straw.
Doctor The last straw?
Patient I feel so ashamed. I should have been able to sort it out myself. I've always coped before.
Doctor So I guess you might be feeling a bit angry and humiliated?
Patient You're damn right. But I suppose I've nothing to lose by being here.
Doctor O.K., well would you mind telling me what's been happening then I can see if your being here makes any sense?
Patient I've just got so terribly low, I can't see any future. I'm sure the cancer is going to eat me away.

OPENING GAMBITS

You should begin the main interview by using a question which reminds the patient that you would like to begin by focusing on his or her presenting problems, for example, "Would you mind beginning by telling me what problems have led to your coming here?". As the patient begins to talk he/she will give several useful cues about apparent or definite problems. After a few minutes you should acknowledge and summarize these cues and then check if there have been any other problems before proceeding with the interview.

Doctor Would you like to tell me what has brought you to hospital today?
Patient I've been feeling ever so run down. I've been sleeping badly. I find myself blowing my top for no reason and I get these terrible panics. I can't understand it. It's not like me at all.

Doctor So you've been feeling run down, had difficulty in sleeping, been blowing your top, and you've had these terrible panics. I'd like to go into each of these in a moment, but are there any other problems that you've noticed?

Patient I've been feeling so miserable; I feel I've fallen into a deep pit. I'm scared that I'm not ever going to be able to climb out. I just don't seem to have any energy. I can't be bothered with anything; I've let the house go to pot. It's so unlike me.

Doctor Anything else you've noticed?

Patient I don't think so.

Doctor Are you sure?

Patient Yes.

ORGANIZING THE INFORMATION

You now have the problem of how best to organize this information and use it in your patient's interest. You should, therefore, again summarize what you have learned so far ("Can I just pause and check that I've heard you correctly? You've been feeling rundown, sleeping badly, blowing your top, getting terrible panics, feeling miserable, have no energy, and you've been letting things go?". Patient: "Yes that's right".) and then give the patient a chance to indicate which problem he or she would like to start with.

Doctor As I explained, I'd now like to go into each of those problems you mentioned. Which would you like to start with?

Patient This feeling so miserable.

DELINEATING THE PROBLEMS

Your task now is to get an exact description of each identified problem. You should so so by encouraging the patient to provide as vivid and accurate a description as possible. The following techniques will help you to do this.

Clarification

With phrases like 'so miserable' it is important that you push the patient a step further and find out what this experience was like.

Doctor You say you felt so miserable – what exactly was that like?
Patient I felt I was enveloped in a black cloud. Everything looked black. I felt I had fallen into a deep pit and could see no way of climbing out. I gave up hope of doing so. Life seemed quite pointless and hopeless.

You will also get closer to your patients' experiences by asking for a detailed example of what they have been experiencing.

Doctor These 'panics' of yours, when was your last one?
Patient Last Wednesday.
Doctor Can you describe exactly what happened?

Doctor You say you were wiped out. Just how were you then?
Patient I was at an absolute standstill. I couldn't be bothered to get up in the mornings. My husband ended up doing the housework. I was too tired to get out of bed. Yet, I couldn't get to sleep and I was off my food.

Such clarifying statements generate further cues about additional problems like sleep disturbance and loss of appetite which also require clarification.

Furthering your understanding

As you clarify the nature of your patient's experiences you may begin to get a clear sense of how your patient really thinks or feels about them. It is important that you test your hypothesis since the patient can then confirm, correct or refute it.

Doctor I get the feeling that you see yourself as on the scrap heap.

Patient I do. I'm no use to anyone as I am. Yet I daren't do more in case I bring on another massive heart attack. (Confirmation with elaboration)

Doctor It sounds as if your recent heart attack was the last straw for you.

Patient No, it wasn't so much the heart attack as learning that I was going to be made redundant. (Correction)

Note that the psychiatrists put their hypotheses in a tentative or 'negotiating style' so that the patients feel able to elaborate further or correct them.

Precision

When information about onsets of key symptoms and timing of potentially relevant events is first presented it is often vague. It may also be biased because of the patients' need to explain their illness in terms of an understandable and acceptable cause. So you should encourage accuracy and precision from the outset.

Doctor When did you first begin to feel anxious?
Patient Sometime last year.
Doctor When last year?
Patient In the summer.
Doctor When exactly in the summer?
Patient August, I think.
Doctor When in August?
Patient I'm not sure.
Doctor Was anything else happening around that time, any key date like a birthday?
Patient Our wedding anniversary was on the 8th of August.
Doctor And when did your anxious feelings begin?
Patient Oh, a few days after I think.

The encouragement of such precision will also lead your patients to take more care to give you an accurate account of their symptoms, feelings and attitudes.

As soon as you sense any inconsistencies you should check these out, otherwise you may remain uncertain about key issues.

Doctor I'm a bit puzzled. You say you got depressed because you were made redundant. But you said you first got depressed last May and you lost your job in September.
Patient Yes, what I meant was that I got even more depressed when I lost my job.

Facilitation

With some patients you may have to actively facilitate their disclosure. You can do this verbally by repeating their last phrase ("hearing voices?") or encouraging them to continue by saying "right", "go on" or "tell me more about it".

Non-verbal facilitation may be done by nodding, making eye contact or smiling, and adopting an attentive posture.

If the patients still appear loath to talk you should acknowledge and explore this.

Doctor You seem to find it difficult to talk to me.
Patient Yes.
Doctor Would you mind telling me why?
Patient I don't know where to start. I feel so confused.
Doctor So confused?
Patient My thoughts aren't making any sense.

Non-verbal cues

As you are talking to your patients they will often give non-verbal cues about possible problems, feelings and attitudes. It is important to note these and acknowledge and clarify them at some point.

Doctor When you mentioned your husband you sounded angry.
Patient Angry. I hate him for what he's done to us.

Doctor You didn't seem to be with me just then, could you tell me what was happening?
Patient Didn't you hear those voices?

Question style

You should try to put your questions singly, simply and in a form which does not bias the answer.

Doctor How has your appetite been?
Patient I haven't any.
Doctor What about your weight?
Patient I've lost over 2 stones.

Control

Once you have got your patient talking about a key problem you must maintain your focus until you have clarified it fully. Otherwise you will move or be moved too soon onto other problems.

Doctor Just how low did you get?
Patient I've been feeling diabolical. Wouldn't you if your wife had gone off with your best friend?
Doctor When did she leave?

This doctor never did establish how low the patient was or that he felt suicidal, for he was side-tracked onto the marital problems.

If you are to stay with a key problem, you should exert control by explaining what you want to focus on and why, and then checking if this is alright.

Doctor Just how low did you get?
Patient Diabolical. Wouldn't you if your wife had gone off with your best friend?
Doctor Yes, it must have been terrible for you. I'd like to ask you more about that in a minute because it's clearly important. But can I just check how low you got?
Patient I got to thinking I might as well shoot myself.

Control is also necessary when you think the patient is getting off the point. Then you should check this and explain what you would like to move on to and why.

Doctor Yes, you've clearly had a lot happening in your family. But how much has that to do with how you are now?
Patient Not that much I suppose.
Doctor In that case can I get back to focusing on how you are now.

At a certain point in an interview you may need to impose your professional agenda, that is areas you have to cover because it seems the best time. If you do this you should make this explicit.

Doctor You've helpfully told me just how depressed you've been in your spirits, and that you've been so low you wanted to kill yourself; can I now ask you some general questions about other things that you might have noticed in relation to your depression?
Patient All right.
Doctor How have you been sleeping?
Patient Not very well.
Doctor How do you mean 'not very well'?
Patient Well, I've been having fitful sleep.
Doctor Can you give me a picture of a typical night? What time do you go to bed?
Patient 10 o'clock.
Doctor And how long is it before you get to sleep?
Patient It takes me at least two to three hours.
Doctor Why is that?
Patient All the dreadful thoughts keep going round in my mind.
Doctor What dreadful thoughts?
Patient That I'm useless and a burden, and that the family would be better off without me.
Doctor And once you've got to sleep how long do you stay asleep?
Patient Oh, I never seem to stay asleep more than an hour or so, I keep waking.
Doctor What time do you finally wake?
Patient Never later than 4 or 5 in the morning.
Doctor How does that compare with before you became depressed?
Patient Oh I used to wake normally at 6.30 or 7.

CLOSING GAMBITS

Once you have elicited the history, it is worth warning your patients that the interview is coming to an end and adding that you would like to summarize what you have learned about their problems. After this summary you should ask "Is there anything else you would like to correct – or add?".

GIVING INFORMATION

Once you have assessed the mental state, made your diagnosis and considered possible treatments, you need to discuss your views with the patient.

You should do this by categorizing what you intend to say and then dealing with each category (for example, what is wrong, why it has happened, and what you plan to do) separately.

Doctor First let me explain what I think happened.
Patient O.K.
Doctor You have developed agorophobia.
Patient I thought so. I've read about it in magazines.

As you deal with each category you should elicit your patients' views and determine if they differ markedly from your own for this could hinder compliance.

Doctor Have you had any thought about treatment?
Patient I don't want any tranquillisers. They just make you dependent. I've enough problems as it is.
Doctor But these antidepressants I mentioned are not tranquillisers and won't lead to dependence. They have a specific action. Would you like me to tell you about this?
Patient Yes, I would.

Finally, you should check if the patient has understood your advice and has any questions.

SELF-MONITORING

You can use a small audiotape recorder to assess your interviewing skills, but increasingly psychiatric tutors are organizing group teaching in interview skills using audio- or videotaped interviews. Most patients will agree to this providing that you explain that it is to help you monitor how you talk to your patients. It will illustrate that you already possess strengths but may also need to improve in certain areas. Continued self-monitoring or group training in interview skills will enable you to determine if you are improving and, in the case of group training, learn from your colleagues as well.

Further reading

Maguire GP (1983) The psychiatric interview. In Kendell RE and Zealley AK, eds. *Companion to Psychiatric Studies, 3rd Edition,* pp.190–204. Edinburgh: Churchill Livingstone

6

Personality and Mental State Examination

Andrew Sims

AIMS OF THE MENTAL STATE EXAMINATION

Medical diagnosis has been based traditionally upon history-taking and examination. In *general medicine* taking the history involves the ears of the doctor, whilst examination implies observation by listening, seeing and touching, and sometimes also smelling! Whilst mental state examination also depends upon observation in other sensory modalities, the emphasis is upon listening – in making inferences from what the patient says. Eliciting psychiatric symptoms is difficult and requires persistence, an ability to communicate, sensitivity to the feelings of the person who is perplexed and distressed, and knowledge of psychiatric disorders. Of course, the mental state is revealed during history-taking, and its evaluation should take into account the social context.

One needs to realise there is conflict of interest between patient and interviewer, and the latter is faced with the problem of having his intentions misunderstood. The patient describes unpleasant experiences that make him feel upset; he wants to get rid of them and hopes that describing his symptoms to the doctor will be the first stage in removing them. He is concerned with *content* – that "my body and lungs are filling up with water and I will drown", or "the Freemasons are sending messages to make me impotent". The doctor, however, is concerned with many things that seem irrelevant to the patient, who may find the doctor's preoccupations irritating and unhelpful. The doctor requires a precise description of the symptoms in terms of their *form*. He wants to know about the patient's development and course through life, about his adjustment to his environment, and about his present emotional state. Our first patient is drowning internally and wants the doctor to deal with the water inside him; the doctor will be more interested in establishing the symptoms and signs of depressive psychosis. Our second patient wants somebody to stop Freemasons from harming him, whilst the doctor will wish to ascertain whether the messages are auditory hallucinations and, if so, of what type.

Each question during the mental state examination should be carefully chosen to reveal specific useful information; knowing everything about the patient is neither valuable nor possible. With each question the doctor should be anticipating what possible answers to that question could come from a reasonable person in this context. A bizarre or unusual response should sensitize him to attempt to clarify the inner experience which has been partly revealed. The doctor should also be looking for the appropriate psychopathological symptoms to make or confirm the diagnosis by *direct questioning.*

The clinical interviewer needs to be careful not to inhibit the patient's answers by imposing psychiatric terminology. A patient experiencing almost continuous auditory hallucinations may reply negatively to the question "Do you hear voices?". He may think of auditory hallucinations as 'messages' which he is receiving in audible form from a source outside his head. It is the nature of the *subjective experience*, and not the precise words used, which carries phenomenological meaning.

In psychiatric examination there is considerable value in deliberately vague questions in the initial stages of enquiry. For example, "Do you sometimes have unusual experiences?". Such questions are less embarrassing than specific interrogation, and can be asked of anyone; they are less directive and allow unexpected material to be revealed. They are useful in pointing out the areas for further and more detailed questioning. The patient should not be exhausted by a long interview; it is better to go back and continue on another day.

[illegible]s has made an important comparison between *understanding*, which is the essential element of psychopathological enquiry, and *explanation*, the normal process of objective scientific investigation. In understanding the psychiatrist uses his own capacity for empathy to reveal precisely the patient's internal, subjective mental state, and how the patient's present experience and behaviour have emerged from previous subjective experiences. In phenomenological enquiry the psychiatrist describes back to the patient what he has ascertained the latter's own experience to be, in such detail and with such empathic understanding that the patient recognizes it as his own.

An important part of the examination of the patient is assessment of the *premorbid, interval* or *usual personality* (Table 6.1). Evaluating premorbid personality solely on the basis of how the patient presents at interview during his illness implies that personality must be relatively consistent despite the vicissitudes of illness and other changes in environment. This is an assumption which is not always justifiable, and where possible an informant should be interviewed. In evaluating the patient for personality characteristics the doctor asks the patient to describe his relationships with other people, his interests and activities. He also studies the way in which the patient reacts to him during interview and he asks the patient to describe himself, his aims and goals.

Table 6.1. A plan for the examination of personality and mental state

Evaluation of usual or premorbid personality

- Description of this individual patient during interview
- Enquiry for specific relevant personality traits
  - effect of these traits upon personal relationships
  - illustration of personality traits in anecdotes from history
- Social relationships
- Activities and interests enjoyed
- Predominant mood
- Character traits
- Attitudes and values
- Initiative and drive
- Fantasy life
- Habits

Appearance and behaviour
- Physical appearance – posture and movement
- Consciousness and attention
- Dress
- Behaviour in interview situation
  - observed at other times

Form of talk
- Rate, quantity
- Continuity, coherence, pauses
- Use of words and syntax
- Non-social speech
- RECORD VERBATIM SAMPLES OF SPEECH

Mood
- Subjective description of mood – in detail
- Objective assessment of mood
- Rapport

Thought content
- Predominant thoughts and mood
  - morbid thoughts – suicidal ideas
- Disturbance of thought processes
- Obsessional ideas or compulsive acts
- Phobias
- Body image

Abnormal beliefs
- Ideas of reference, misinterpretations
- Overvalued ideas
- Delusions

Abnormal perceptions
- Pain
- Illusions
- Hallucinations
- Depersonalization and derealization
- Other abnormal perceptions

Cognitive function
- Orientation
- Long-term memory
- Registration and short-term memory
- Immediate memory
- Attention and concentration
- General information
- Current affairs
- Abstract thinking
- Intelligence

Insight

Reaction to patient

ASSESSMENT OF PERSONALITY AND PERSONALITY DISORDER

For clinical description of personality disorder a typology is usually used. That contained in ICD-9 is recommended, not because it is faultless, but because if general application is made of this scheme a consensus will emerge on the use of terms. In Table 6.2 the types of personality disorder in ICD-9 are compared with the American DSM-III.

Table 6.2. Comparison of Personality Types in ICD-9 and DSM-III

ICD-9		DSM-III
301.0	Paranoid	Paranoid
301.1	Affective	
301.2	Schizoid	Schizoid Schizotypal
301.3	Explosive	
301.4	Anankastic	Compulsive
301.5	Hysterical	Histrionic
301.6	Asthenic	Dependent
301.7	Asocial	Antisocial
301.8	'Other'	Narcissistic Avoidant Borderline Passive–aggressive Atypical, mixed, or other

Personality assessment consists of looking for the predominant traits; a decision as to whether personality is fundamentally normal or abnormal; and if abnormal, an evaluation of what abnormality is present. Personality is that part of a person that makes him individual, that is different from other people; it is revealed by characteristic behaviour and is useful in that it predicts future responses. Categorization into *normal* and *abnormal* personality is based upon the use of the word *normal* in a statistical sense; that is, a characteristic of personality is normal if common to the majority, and abnormal if present only in the minority, irrespective of value judgement. Abnormal personality therefore has some characteristics developed or under-developed to such an extent as to be quantitatively different from the mass of the population. It is manifest in certain patterns of behaviour which are of clinical importance. However, many people will show a combination of different types of personality.

Personality disorder is present when the abnormality of personality causes either the patient himself to suffer or other people to suffer. Personality abnormality is part of the individual's constitution, but whether or not this manifests as personality disorder depends to a considerable extent on the social context; for example, abnormality which in one situation may be deemed criminal psychopathy may in another be welcomed as the characteristics of a creative political revolutionary.

The ability to differentiate between normal and abnormal has to be learnt as a clinical skill. Assessment of personality has not become useful clinically until it is effective in predicting behaviour. For a satisfactory assessment of personality it is important to include objective observations of personality characteristics by the doctor, verbatim statements from the patient of his aims and goals, and how he feels about himself, a comment on the quality of his social relationships, and a *summary* of the personality in terms of predominant traits, whether personality is abnormal, and if so whether this amounts to personality disorder. Painting the picture in description and defining the type are both equally important.

Social relationships are assessed by such questions as:

How does he relate to his family? Is he detached or over-dependent? What sort of friendships does he form, with what sort of people, and are they close-knit or superficial, with an exclusive few or an unlimited crowd? How do his interests and leisure activities involve him with others; social or solitary; structured or informal? How does he relate to bosses, workmates and employees? Is he a leader or a follower, an organizer, an isolant, pliant or truculent, cooperative or clubable? What are his sexual preferences and orientation in social relationships?

Information concerning interests and activities is sought. If he is interested in sport, is it as participant or observer? His interests in films and literature are relevant, as are the societies to which he belongs and his religious beliefs, affiliations and practices.

Enquiry is made of his predominant moods and whether these are fluctuating or stable, responsive to precipitants or endogenous. His character traits are described, as are his attitudes and values, his views about himself and his body. His general level of drive and energy are evaluated. Enquiry is made of fantasy life, the frequency and duration of daydreams and their content; whether these are realistic plans for the future or unattainable 'castles in the air'.

Detailed enquiry should be made about habits such as smoking, alcohol intake and patterns of eating. The aim is to have an understanding of his functioning as a whole person. Allocating the patient to a personality type without taking into account the infinite variability of different individuals is unsatisfactory, and a full description should always precede categorization. However, assessing the predominance of different characteristics and then deciding on the personality type has some predictive value. A brief summary of predominant traits for different personality types is included in Table 6.3.

Table 6.3. Types of Personality (based upon ICD-9)

301.0	Paranoid	misconstrues others' personal rights, jealousy, self-importance, self-reference, fanatical, litiginous
301.1	Affective	pronounced mood lifelong: depressive or elated, cyclothymic, anxious
301.2	Schizoid	withdrawal, coolness and detachment
301.3	Explosive	liability to intemperate outbursts of mood
301.4	Anankastic	insecurity, doubt, conscientiousness, perfectionism, rigidity
301.5	Hysterical	shallow, labile affect, appreciation craving, theatricality, sexual immaturity
301.6	Asthenic	passive compliance, inadequacy, lack of vigour
301.7	Asocial	lack of feeling for others, callous, cold, rejects social norms, irresponsible, does not learn from experience

FRAMEWORK FOR DESCRIBING MENTAL STATE PHENOMENA

It is a good habit to make observations under all the headings listed below for all patients in this or any other appropriate sequence so that important areas are not omitted. The *mental state examination* is not confined to asking specific questions. Visual observations are extremely important, as are noticing unusual responses to questions during history-taking and the responses of the patient to distractions outside the interview room, and so on. The importance of recording verbatim remarks of the patient cannot be stressed too much.

Appearance and behaviour

Observation is used for making clinical judgements; this implies that the observer will understand the significance of abnormalities in appearance and behaviour and how they relate to different conditions. Ethnicity, physique, dress, make-up, length of hair, cleanliness, and so on are noted. Does the patient look ill? Is he alert, orientated, fully conscious, or fluctuating in his mental state? Are there any behavioural or neurological abnormalities present on observation? What is the quality of non-verbal communication in terms of posture, gesture, facial expression and attitude to the observer? Are there any indicators of psychiatric symptomatology such as tics, catatonic movements, behaviour suggestive of hallucinatory perceptions, feeding or eating disorders, restlessness or akathisia? What is the level of activity in terms of retardation or excitement, distractibility?

If the patient is mute, observed behaviour is the only source of clinical information and will then be even more important. However, the value of observation should be stressed also for those patients who do speak. It may be useful to corroborate the patient's complaints, to make more clear the degree of emotional involvement he has in his symptoms, or sometimes to contradict his statement.

Form of talk

Talking reveals thinking and so listening to the patient is usually the most important part of the mental state examination. Is speech unusual in rate or quantity? Does the patient talk volubly and easily or in taciturn monosyllables? Does he just answer questions or speak spontaneously? Is there evidence of pressure of talk, circumstantiality or, alternatively, slowness or silence?

It is important to note if speech is appropriate to the social situation and coherent. Are there pauses in conversation suggestive of thought blocking? Does the patient ask questions in an appropriate way and keep to the topic of conversation?

Note is taken of the patient's use of grammar and of words, and of the association between sentences. *Neologisms* may be produced, or existing words or phrases may be used in an idiosyncratic way. The abnormalities of grammar, if consistent, should be noted and abnormal speech recorded verbatim. Non-social speech includes grunts, mutterings, and so on.

Mood

There are three aspects for exploration: *subjective* and *objective* description of mood and measurement of *rapport*. The subjective description of affect is much more subtle than just depression or elation; these nuances require clarification. Mood should be studied in terms of direction (depression or elation), consistency (stable or labile), appropriateness, amplitude, and the degree of discrepancy between subjective description and objective observation.

Assessment of the patient's mood is not, and should not be, totally objective; it involves the use of empathy, the ability to put oneself in the patient's position in order to understand what his current affect must be like. The interviewer picks up and records verbal and visual cues (monotonous voice, furrowed brow) and comes to the judgement "If I felt how my patient looks, speaks and acts, I would feel profoundly depressed; on observation he is depressed".

Rapport assesses the patient's ability to communicate his feelings to another person. For this the interviewer, from previous experience and objectivity, needs to regard himself as a 'constant rapport maker' measuring the patient's capacity to establish rapport.

Thought content

Here one is attempting to demonstrate the most prominent content of thinking; what occupies the patient's mind. This will include enquiry for morbid thoughts and suicidal ideas. Such abnormalities of thinking as obsessions and compulsions, ruminations both depressive and obsessional, phobias and overvalued ideas should be demonstrated phenomenologically, and this demands a basic knowledge of psychopathology.

Obsessions or *compulsions* should be looked for, bearing in mind the following characteristics: the thought or behaviour is repetitive, regarded as being initiated by the self but at the same time senseless, unnecessary or unrewarding, resisted but unsuccessfully. *Phobias* are unreasonable fears that come to dominate the patient's consciousness; they are usually volunteered early in the interview.

Ideas about the body should be explored. Do the patient's views about health and illness amount to *hypochondriasis*? Is the complaint about an individual organ indicative of *dysmorphophobia?* Is there a generalized body image disorder?

Abnormal beliefs

The great danger here is that the doctor will only *hear* what *he thinks* the patient means to say, as occurs in ordinary social settings, rather than allow the patient to express his beliefs in their stark *un-understandability*. Ideas of guilt, hypochondriacal, nihilistic and self-referrent ideas and overvalued ideas need to be distinguished from delusions. Delusions (and hallucinations) may not be volunteered by the patient as symptoms because they are not experienced subjectively as being different from usual experience.

Careful probes may be required to expose delusions: "Do you sometimes feel people are against you in some way?". This general question will then require more detailed supplementary investigation. Delusional systems may be revealed on further questioning. Delusions of control (passivity experiences) will often only become apparent upon direct enquiry.

Abnormal perceptions

This should include enquiry about external sensation, internal experience and the interpretations the patients makes about them. Depersonalization, derealization and related phenomena may be revealed at this stage. Patients have great difficulty in describing depersonalization despite it being very frequent. They do not have words for the symptom; they feel they must be unique and that if they admit to so bizarre and troublesome a complaint the doctor will think they are mad. If the patient complains of *pain*, this should be explored in detail.

Hallucination, which usually has pathological significance, needs to be distinguished from other abnormalities of perception such as *illusion, vivid imagery* and *pseudohallucination*. The sensory modality is important and auditory hallucinations need to be explored in their detailed psychopathology: inside or outside the head? One voice or more than one voice? Speaking in the third person or not? – and so on.

Cognitive function

Clinical examination differs from psychometry in that there is no intention to produce a score. The doctor is concerned with abnormality; is there a discrepancy between what is found and what could reasonably be expected from this person when in health?

Orientation is tested with respect to time, place and person. Disorientation in *time* occurs earliest in an illness; it should be tested for by asking the date, including month and year, the day of the week, the time of day, duration of passage of time. Orientation in *space* is best tested by asking the patient to find his way in a known environment; for *person* is tested by the interviewer introducing himself at the beginning with his name and designation, and asking for this information at this point in the examination.

Long-term memory disturbance is revealed during history-taking but requires confirmation from an informant. *Registration* and *short-term memory* are tested by asking the patient to repeat a name and address (registration and immediate memory), and then recall it after 15 minutes (short-term memory). A rough score can be given: Mr(1) John(2) Robinson(3), 27(4) Grove(5) Avenue(6), Nottingham(7). Digit span forwards is a useful further test for *immediate memory*. It is important not to emphasize certain digits, nor to break the number into sequences. For this test the interviewer compares observed result with expected result (an accountant would be expected to score higher than a hospital cleaner).

A two-sentence test is useful, as not only does it test memory, but it may also provoke *perseveration*. The patient is told that he will be given two sentences to repeat; he is asked to repeat the first after he has been given it, and then similarly the second; he is then asked to repeat the first again, and then the second:

1. "The river passes by with a soft murmuring sound."
2. "The cricket match was won in the very last over."

Accurate reproduction may also be tested by using one of the Babcock sentences, for example:

"One thing a nation must have to become rich and great is a large, secure supply of wood."

The number of repetitions needed for accurate reproduction is recorded.

Attention and *concentration* may be tested by asking the patient to give a series of digits in reverse order, or to recite the days of the week in reverse order. The serial 7s test, subtracting in 7s from 100, may be used. The number of errors and the time taken are noted.

Enquiry is made for *general information* and *current affairs*. Names of monarchs or prime ministers are asked, going backwards in time. The patient is asked for capital cities of countries. However, many answers may reveal educational rather than intellectual deficiency. Knowledge of current affairs is sought, especially concentrating on areas in which the patient has already expressed an interest.

Abstract thinking is tested by asking for the meaning of proverbs; again educational deficit may interfere. It is preferable to use proverbs that the patient does not know well, as one is not trying to test memory. Asking for the differences between such pairs as ice and glass, child and dwarf, may be used.

After completing the tests of cognitive function it should be possible to estimate the intellectual performance in interview and compare it with presumed performance from the history *(intelligence)*.

Insight

This is the ability of the patient to understand his own experiences, to realise that he is ill, and in what way he is ill. The patient's view of his mental state and his illness is compared with their objective assessment. When insight is diminished it is usually partially so, and it is important to describe in what way. Statements such as 'intact' or 'absent' should not be used.

Reaction to patient

How the interviewer is affected by the patient may indicate how others are affected. The interviewer describes his feelings (e.g. anger, irritation, sadness, concern, suspicion) and how he controlled them.

In the mental state examination and in the assessment of personality, each item should be summarized in terms of normality or abnormality. If there is abnormality, the significance of this should be demonstrated and its relevance to the final diagnosis; thus "garrulous, voluble speech at a great rate" might be summarized as *pressure of talk,* which suggests the diagnosis of *mania.* The aim of the mental state examination is to establish the diagnosis, and this should be borne in mind throughout.

Further reading

American Psychiatric Association (1980) *Diagnostic and Statistical Manual of Mental Disorders, 3rd Edition.* Washington: American Psychiatric Association

Jaspers K (1962). *General Psychopathology.* Translated from German 7th Edition by Hoenig J and Hamilton MW. Manchester: Manchester University Press

Leff JP and Isaacs AD (1978) *Psychiatric Examination in Clinical Practice.* Oxford: Blackwell

Sims ACP (1987) *Symptoms in the Mind: An Introduction to Descriptive Psychopathology.* Eastbourne: Baillière Tindall

Strub RL and Black FW (1977) *The Mental Status Examination in Neurology.* Philadelphia: FA Davis Company

Tyrer P and Alexander J (1979) Classification of personality disorder. *British Journal of Psychiatry 135:* 163–167

Withers E and Hinton J (1971) Three forms of the clinical tests of the sensorium and their reliability. *British Journal of Psychiatry 119:* 1–8

World Health Organisation (1977) *International Classification of Diseases, Injuries and Causes of Death, 9th Revision.* Geneva: WHO

7

Physical Examination

E. Szabadi

Physical examination is an essential part of everyday medical practice, and as psychiatry is a branch of medicine, it cannot be practised without the competent physical examination. The purpose of this chapter is to give some guidelines concerning both the routine examination of patients and also the examination of special categories of patients.

THE IMPORTANCE OF PHYSICAL EXAMINATION

There are several reasons why physical examination is essential in everyday psychiatric practice. (1) The psychiatric illness may be secondary to an underlying physical illness. This is the case when few dispute the importance of physical examination, and it would be deplorable to overlook an identifiable physical abnormality which plays a causative role in the psychiatric syndrome (e.g. the patient who has brain tumour and presents with depression or paranoid psychosis, or the patient with thyrotoxicosis presenting with an anxiety state or manic psychosis). (2) The psychiatric illness presents in a patient who also has a physical disease or abnormality. Although there may not be a causal relationship between the physical and psychiatric syndromes, the physical illness is likely to play a pathoplastic role in the genesis of the psychiatric picture (e.g. anxiety state in a patient with Crohn's disease; depression in a patient with bronchial asthma). The presence of the physical disorder may also modify plans for management (e.g. contraindication of certain drugs) and the assessment of prognosis. (3) The psychiatric illness results in physical symptoms and signs. Many psychiatric illnesses produce more-or-less characteristic bodily changes, e.g. movement disorders associated with schizophrenia; emaciation, lanugo hair, acrocyanosis in anorexia nervosa; autonomic changes (tachycardia, sweating) in anxiety states; scars associated with self-inflicted injuries in some cases of personality disorder and mental subnormality. (4) The underlying disorder results in both physical and mental signs. This applies to some cases of mental subnormality (e.g. Down's syndrome, phenylketonuria, tuberous sclerosis, Sturge-Weber syndrome). (5) The drug prescribed for a psychiatric condition results in physical symptoms and signs (e.g. motor side-effects of antipsychotics, orthostatic hypotension produced by monoamine oxidase inhibitors, tachycardia produced by tricyclic antidepressants). (6) The patient complains of physical symptoms (e.g. pain, breathlessness, odd bodily sensations, alterations to the appearance of the body), but there is no identifiable underlying physical abnormality. Many of these patients are referred to the psychiatrist by other doctors, often after numerous investigations and/or surgical operations have been done, and often with the label of 'hysteria' or 'hypochondriasis'. It is essential for the psychiatrist to examine these patients thoroughly, not because it is likely that he might discover a physical disease overlooked by the neurologists or surgeons, but because he has to demonstrate to the patient that he is also a doctor who takes the patient and his complaints seriously. (7) Physical signs may shed light on the aetiology or some pathogenic factors (e.g. smell of alcohol on breath; drug injection sites; bruises indicating violence; constricted pupils indicating opiate abuse; dilated pupils indicating amphetamine abuse, etc.). (8) Patients who have psychiatric 'diagnostic labels' (e.g. chronic schizophrenia, dementia, personality disorder) attached to them are not immune to physical disease. Indeed, complaints arising in such (often long-stay) patients may be attributed to the psychiatric illness and the newly developed physical illness overlooked. Therefore psychiatric patients with new complaints should be examined physically.

Thus, it is apparent that only a few psychiatric patients could be excused of a thorough physical examination. Since it is very difficult to identify these patients before a physical examination is carried out, it seems to be reasonable to examine most, if not all, patients referred to the psychiatrist. However, the finding of no abnormality on physical examination does not mean that the examination was superfluous: very often negative findings are just as informative as positive ones and the examination may facilitate the doctor-patient relationship.

CARRYING OUT THE PHYSICAL EXAMINATION

Physical examination of the patient relies on the application of a number of basic classical clinical skills (inspection, auscultation, palpation, tapping), and involves the use of only a few simple instruments (reflex hammer, sphygmomanometer, ophthalmoscope, tuning fork, etc.). Most psychiatric units have special examination rooms so that the examination can be carried out in privacy, in a thorough, systematic, unhurried fashion. It is helpful if a nurse can be present to assist with undressing/dressing if the patient is physically infirm or uncooperative, and also as a chaperone (see also p.201). Examination findings should be recorded immediately to ensure that nothing is forgotten.

In-patients should be examined on the day of admission. This usually takes place after the history has been taken, relatives interviewed, and mental state assessed (but see also p.201). If the patient is exhausted by the end of the interview, it is reasonable to allow the patient to settle on the ward, and conduct the 'physical' a couple of hours later. This order of procedure helps the psychiatrist to have some idea of the psychiatric problem before he examines the patient physically.

Out-patients are usually not examined routinely in psychiatric clinics. Unfortunately it is not practicable for clinics with heavy case-loads. Patients referred by their general practitioners or hospital doctors usually have already had a physical examination in the recent past, and the results of this are communicated to the psychiatrist. In some cases (see p.79), however, it is impossible to forfeit the physical examination. Most out-patient departments are equipped with an examination room for this purpose.

Day-patients and *long-stay in-patients* should always be examined if they present with new complaints or signs (see above). It is more difficult, however, to set a rule stating how frequently such patients should undergo *routine* physical examinations in the absence of new complaints or obvious clinical deterioration. A bi-monthly routine physical examination seems to be a reasonable practice.

EXAMINING PARTICULAR TYPES OF PATIENT

The patient with signs of alcohol or drug intoxication

Patients under the acute influence of alcohol or other psychoactive drugs are often seen in the casualty department or at a police station. In the case of alcohol intoxication the patient usually smells of alcohol and shows typical features (some clouding of consciousness, psychomotor agitation or retardation, garrulousness, hostility or over-friendliness, cerebellar ataxia, vomiting, conjunctival injection). However, research has shown that the diagnosis of alcohol intoxication on clinical grounds is unreliable (see p.97). Intoxicated patients may be uncooperative with the examination, and detailed examination may not be possible until the effects of alcohol or drugs have worn off. In an intoxicated state, the patient may have sustained some injuries which can be uncovered only by a thorough physical examination. The intoxicated patient may suffer from various physical or psychiatric disorders which may be detected only by examination and observation. Intoxication with drugs other than alcohol (barbiturates, amphetamine, heroin, cannabis, psilocybin, LSD) can result in alterations in the level of consciousness and/or psychomotor tempo rendering the patient uncooperative (see below). There may be some pointers in the direction of intoxication by certain drugs: slurred speech, ataxia, nystagmus, drowsiness may indicate barbiturates; dilated pupils, psychomotor agitation, increased sympathetic activity may suggest amphetamine; constricted pupils, emotional indifference, together with injection sites may be indicative of opiate abuse. However, in cases of poly-drug abuse clinical signs may be confusing.

The uncooperative patient

There are two major categories of uncooperative patients: patients with and patients without an alteration of consciousness. The alteration in the level of consciousness may vary along a continuum from a relatively mild clouding of consciousness (as in organic confusional states and deliria) through semi-coma to coma. While patients presenting with an organic confusional state or delirium show a fluctuating level of consciousness and maintain some rapport with the environment, and thus may cooperate to some extent with the examination, the comatose patient is unresponsive to external stimuli and thus completely uncooperative. In delirium the clouding of consciousness is usually accompanied by extreme psychomotor agitation rendering the patient very difficult to examine.

There are several features of the mental state that may render patients, whose level of consciousness is unaltered, uncooperative: (1) stupor, (2) retardation, (3) hyperactivity, (4) delusions, (5) impaired attention, (6) hostility, (7) cognitive-impairment. In *stupor* the patient is akinetic and mute with relative preservation of conscious awareness. This syndrome can be due to organic causes (lesions in the diencephalon and upper brain stem: 'akinetic mutism'), may be the feature of a functional psychosis (e.g. depressive or catatonic stupor), or of a dissociative state (hysterical stupor). The physical examination will become especially difficult if the stupor is accompanied by negativism. Severe *retardation* can be a feature of depression; in extreme forms it can reach the intensity of depressive stupor. Hypokinesia and lack of spontaneity can also be the features of the frontal lobe syndrome; these patients, however, usually follow instructions and cooperate with the examination. The *hyperactivity* of the manic syndrome can disrupt the patient's normal activities and seriously impair cooperation with the examination. *Delusions* of various kinds can result in lack of cooperation: delusions of persecution may result in suspiciousness, hostility or aggressive behaviour; delusions of grandeur may convince the patient that a medical examination is a trivial or unnecessary affair. *Impaired attention*, as in the manic syndrome, may result in lack of cooperation, even in the absence of disruptive hyperactivity. *Hostility* may result from suspiciousness or delusions. The *cognitive impairment* seen in patients with mental subnormality or dementia may result in difficulties in grasping the doctor's instructions.

If the patient does not cooperate with the examination, assistance from nurses or other doctors will become especially important. Actively hostile or aggressive patients often cooperate if there are several members of staff present. In some cases, it may be impossible to proceed with the examination until the patient's extreme psychomotor agitation is reduced by the administration of a tranquillizer; one single intramuscular injection of droperidol (10mg) may be effective. It is always necessary to undress the patient in order to inspect the whole body and to ascertain the integrity and motility of the limbs. Many parts of the medical and neurological examination can be carried out without the patient's active cooperation. It is more difficult to proceed, however, if the patient is actively resistant; in such cases, it may help to postpone the detailed examination for a few hours, or even until the following day: patients often give up their active resistance after they have settled on the ward and developed some trust in the staff.

Organic psychiatric disorders

The physical examination is of particular importance when the psychiatric syndrome is thought to be secondary to some abnormality of the central nervous system due to some intra- or extracranial pathology. The *general inspection* of the patient may yield some important diagnostic pointers. Thus characteristic changes in the size and shape of the body may indicate psychiatrically relevant endocrine disorders (e.g. acromegaly, Cushing's syndrome, Klinefelter's syndrome). Pallor of the skin may indicate anaemia, kidney disease or myxoedema, and jaundice can be indicative of liver disease. Some skin lesions are pathognomic of psychiatrically relevant diseases, e.g. butterfly-shaped facial erythema in lupus erythematosus, photosensitivity and hyperpigmentation in acute porphyria, adenoma sebaceum in tuberous sclerosis, naevus flammeus in Sturge-Weber syndrome. Muscular twitchings can occur in uraemia, electrolyte disturbance (e.g. lithium intoxication) and hypoglycaemia; choreiform movements can be indicative of Huntington's disease. The *neurological examination* is of particular importance in detecting intracranial pathology: meningeal signs and signs of raised intracranial pressure on the ocular fundi can be indicative of intracranial inflammation, haemorrhage or tumour, whereas abnormalities in the functioning of the cranial nerves, motor and sensory systems can help to pinpoint focal lesions. Examination of the *cardiovascular* and *respiratory systems*, and of the *abdomen* may help to detect some extracranial pathology which may lead either to cerebral hypoxia or metabolic changes affecting brain function.

The patient suffering from an organic psychiatric disorder often falls into the category of the 'uncooperative patient' (see p.83): alteration of consciousness, general cognitive impairment and/or alteration in psychomotor tempo may impair cooperation. The impairment of cooperation may be partial and rather specific in cases of localized lesions of the neocortex: lesions of the frontal lobe can result in disinhibition or psychomotor retardation, parietal lesions can lead to dressing apraxia, and lesions of the temporal lobe can produce impairment of short-term memory rendering cooperation difficult. A full neuropsychological examination is necessary in these cases.

Sexual disorders

Male sexual inadequacy can be due to a variety of organic causes. Inspection of the genitals may reveal testicular atrophy, loss of pubic hair, deformities of the cavernous bodies or hypospadias and rectal examination may reveal prostatic disease. General inspection of the body may reveal endocrine abnormalities, e.g. Cushing's syndrome, Addison's disease, acromegaly, myxoedema, Klinefelter's syndrome. Gynecomastia may be associated with Klinefelter's syndrome, or be the result of increased prolactin secretion as in hypophyseal prolactinoma or as a side-effect of antipsychotic medication. The neurological examination may reveal spinal cord lesions associated with impotence; signs of peripheral neuropathy (muscular atrophy, sensory loss) over the lower extremities may be indicative of neuropathy in the pelvic plexus, resulting in impotence. Hypertension and signs of atherosclerosis may suggest an impairment of the blood supply to the cavernous bodies. In *transsexual patients* inspection of the genitals may reveal signs of self-mutilation which may have bearing on the course of further management. In *female patients* with sexual problems a full gynaecological examination is necessary; such an examination may detect an intact hymen, pregnancy or venereal disease, and is essential in assessing vaginismus and/or dyspareunia.

Mental handicap

General inspection may reveal abnormalities of the size and shape of the body or parts of it associated with mental subnormality (e.g. acrocephaly, Down's syndrome), thwarted growth, malnutrition, accidental and self-inflicted injuries. The appearance of the patient may be indicative of some specific disorder, e.g. pallor and café-au-lait patches of phenylketonuria, adenoma sebaceum of tuberous sclerosis, naevus flammeus on the face of Sturge-Weber syndrome, injuries resulting from self-mutilation of Lesch-Nyhan syndrome. The neurological examination can detect brain damage, and is especially important in the assessment of the degree of handicap and in the construction of a plan for management. Examination of the cardiovascular system can reveal malformations of the heart and large vessels characteristic of the 'rubella syndrome'. Mentally handicapped patients may suffer from acquired illnesses (e.g. infections, injuries) and the physical examination is essential in detecting these. The mentally handicapped patient may not cooperate fully with the examination (see p.83), and therefore the examination requires special skill and perseverance from the doctor.

Patients with a history of excessive drinking

Long-term excessive alcohol consumption can affect many organ systems of the body. General inspection can reveal emaciation due to malnutrition and chronic gastritis; ascites, jaundice, spider naevi, lack of pubic hair, testicular atrophy resulting from liver failure; oedema resulting from hypoproteinaemia, liver failure or beri-beri due to thiamine deficiency. The neurological examination can detect nystagmus and ophthalmoplegia (especially paralysis of conjugate gaze) characteristic of Wernicke's encephalopathy; ataxia associated with cerebellar atrophy, cerebral atrophy, Wernicke's encephalopathy or Marchiafava-Bignami disease; tremor (regularly rhythmic static: alcohol withdrawal; coarse-flapping: liver failure); loss of sensation, reflexes, muscle power in the extremities due to peripheral neuropathy. Cardiovascular examination can reveal cardiomegaly due to cardiomyopathy or beri-beri, often with associated signs of cardiac failure.

Patients with a history of drug abuse

The long-term abuse of drugs other than alcohol has relatively little effect on different organ systems of the body. Cocaine-sniffers characteristically develop a perforation of the nasal septum; opiate abusers may present with the consequences of repeated non-sterile intravenous injections (phlebitis, abscesses) or of serum hepatitis (jaundice, enlarged liver); solvent abusers often have a characteristic rash around the nose and mouth. These signs can be important in confirming the suspicion of drug abuse in a patient. There are no specific physical signs associated with the long-term abuse of amphetamine, LSD or cannabis.

Patients with side-effects of psychotropic drugs

Although patients often complain of the subjective experiences associated with the side-effects of drugs, often only the physical examination can detect or verify unwanted bodily changes produced by a particular drug. General inspection can reveal obesity associated with medication with phenothiazines, tricyclic antidepressants or lithium, and ankle oedema developing on lithium medication. Skin lesions due to drugs are allergic reactions, jaundice, photosensitivity or hyperpigmentation. A stooping posture is characteristic of antipsychotic-induced Parkinsonism, and a general restlessness ('inability to sit still') of neuroleptic-induced akathisia and tricyclic antidepressant withdrawal. Changes in muscle tone can be observed in some patients: cogwheel rigidity in antipsychotic-induced Parkinsonism and spasticity in dystonic reactions. Involuntary movements are frequent complications: (1) tremor (a fine static tremor on lithium medication, a coarse-flapping tremor in lithium intoxication, and a resting tremor in antipsychotic-induced Parkinsonism); (2) acute dystonic reactions sometimes limited to one part of the body such as the muscles of the neck and shoulders, or the pharynx so that the tongue protrudes and the patient cannot swallow, and oculogyric crises associated with some potent antipsychotics, especially butyrophenones; (3) chorea (both orofacial and whole body chorea) in tardive dyskinesia. There may be changes in the cardiovascular system: orthostatic hypotension in patients medicated with neuroleptics, tricyclic antidepressants and MAOIs; hypertension as part of the 'cheese reaction' on MAOI medication; tachycardia in patients treated with tricyclic antidepressants.

Further reading

Bickerstaff ER (1980) *Neurological Examination in Clinical Practice.* Oxford: Blackwell

Cooper AJ (1986) Advances in the assessment of organic causes of impotence. *British Journal of Hospital Medicine 36:* 186–192

Lishman WA (1978) *Organic Psychiatry.* Oxford: Blackwell

Macleod J (1979) *Clinical Examination.* Edinburgh: Churchill Livingstone

Morgan WS and Engel GL (1969) *The Clinical Approach to the Patient.* Philadelphia: WB Saunders

— 8 —

Investigations

P. J. McKenna

In the functional illnesses that make up the bulk of psychiatric referrals, physical investigations are, by definition, negative, and psychological tests, with minor exceptions, have not yet established themselves as aids to diagnosis. In the various disorders subsumed under the term 'organic', both physical and psychological investigations may play a decisive role in diagnosis, but here considerable sophistication is necessary if their use is not to be indiscriminate.

The term 'functional' in psychiatry refers to disorders where there is no evidence for an organic brain dysfunction, either acutely, in the form of an impairment of consciousness, or chronically, as global intellectual deterioration. Organic disorders, in their most important sense, refer to illnesses where a physical disorder affects the brain to disrupt mental function globally. If the onset is relatively abrupt the presentation is one of an acute confusional state. If insidious, the picture is usually that of dementia. Organic disorders produce, as their pathognomonic signs, impairments in intellect, judgement and grasp, although any organic state may be complicated by functional-type symptoms presumed to be 'released' by the cerebral insult. The term organic is also legitimately applied to the uncommon clinical instances where a distinct physical disorder induces psychiatric symptoms which are unaccompanied by confusion or intellectual deterioration and so are indistinguishable from a functional illness. Such cases are usually referred to as *symptomatic* or *secondary*.

In practice, psychiatric illnesses usually segregate themselves into those which are clearly functional and those which are just as clearly organic. Their investigation is relatively straightforward, and is discussed under the heading of *routine investigations of psychiatric patients.* In a minority of cases first diagnosed as functional, the possibility of an organic basis, either symptomatic, confusional or dementing, becomes raised. Evaluation of such states is more complicated and discussed here under *further investigation of psychiatric patients.*

ROUTINE INVESTIGATION OF PSYCHIATRIC PATIENTS

Functional disorders

Physical investigations

The majority of general adult psychiatric patients present with illnesses that appear functional clinically, and which in the long run turn out to reveal no evidence of occult physical disorder. The goal of physical investigations in such patients is therefore one of *screening*, to rule out any possible medical conditions which could conceivably be contributing to the clinical picture, but might go undetected on physical examination. The yield of positive results is in general extremely low. No investigation is indispensible, and the usefulness of all of them has been contested at one time or another. The following list of tests represents a scheme that would not be considered controversial in most departments. They are designed for use in acutely ill patients admitted to in-patient care and would be suitable for cases of schizophrenia, manic-depressive psychosis or major depressive disorders. Judgement should be exercised over their use in re-admissions, and, by and large, they are not necessary in out-patients. Investigations necessary before treatments like ECT or lithium are discussed on pages 183 and 175 respectively.

Routine urinalysis Ward or 'side room' testing of urine for sugar, protein, ketones, blood, bile products and pH is often neglected in psychiatric units. It ought to be carried out before ECT (see p.183) in view of the possible consequences of overlooking a condition such as diabetes.

Routine biochemistry (urea and electrolytes plus liver function tests or automated profile) Unless the patient has some co-existent physical disease, urea and electrolytes rarely show anything other than spurious abnormalities. Liver function tests are useful for adding documentation to alcohol abuse but are rarely, if ever, the only manifestation of this. However, these tests are so cheap that their use has become a part of routine psychiatric practice and only academic or economic purists would advise against their use.

Routine haematology (full blood count plus erythrocyte sedimentation rate or plasma viscosity) The primary justification for this is the same as above. In addition, a raised mean cell volume (MCV) is a sensitive index of excessive alcohol intake and may be the only pointer to excess which is denied by the patient. A raised ESR or PV is occasionally the first indication of underlying organic pathology, notably connective tissue disorders, but, more often than not, follow-up leads nowhere.

Chest and skull X-ray Chest radiography often reveals pathology, but this is invariably irrelevant to the psychiatric diagnosis. Like biochemical and haematological analysis, however, it is a routine part of admission to hospital, can almost be considered part of the physical examination, and occasionally reveals abnormalities which, though coincidental, have important implications for the patient. Skull X-ray is one of the more contentious routine psychiatric investigations. However there is no doubt that radiologically detectable cranial lesions are at least twice as common among psychiatric patients as in the general population and that positive results with diagnostic and therapeutic implications are occasionally seen.

Serology for syphilis (WR and VDRL) This remains, in the view of many psychiatrists, an essential investigation. Cases of general paralysis are still seen, and when they occur this always seems to be in patients in whom the diagnosis has not been considered.

Other investigations Other investigations, notably thyroid function tests, electroencephalography, and serum B_{12} and folate levels are carried out on all new admissions in a few centres; they cannot, however, be considered routine. The trainee should be guided by the policy of his consultant in their use. It seems likely that at some point in the future computerized tomography or other brain imaging techniques will become more or less standard on all patients with major psychiatric illness, but this day is still a long way off. The use of the dexamethasone suppression test is one of several current attempts to identify biological markers of psychiatric disorder. It has not, unfortunately, achieved the sensitivity and specificity required for routine clinical use. A number of analogous procedures are presently under development and may ultimately enter psychiatric practice.

Psychological investigations

Despite numerous attempts, no psychological tool has as yet established itself a place in diagnosis of functional psychiatric disorders. None of the numerous available tests can, therefore, be considered routine, and on the whole the trainee will not be expected to use them. A classification of currently used psychological investigations and some brief statements about their use can be made as follows:

Diagnostic instruments These include the Present State Examination (PSE) in Britain and the Schedule for Affective Disorders and Schizophrenia (SADS) used in the USA. They consist of detailed inventories of questions from which a number of psychiatric diagnoses can be established, according to pre-determined criteria. Their principal use is in research, in particular for standardization of diagnosis in psychosis. As they can only be carried out by an interviewer trained in their use, they have little routine clinical application.

Rating scales These consist mainly of interviewer and self-rates questionnaires of manic, depressive and anxiety symptoms. Examples include the observer rated Montgomery-Åsberg scale and Manchester scales and the self-rated Hospital Anxiety and Depression scale of Zigmond and Snaith. Other scales in common use measure global mental state, general behaviour on the ward and so on. Such investigations are short, easy to master and very useful for monitoring a patient's progress and response to treatment. They are, however, no substitute for clinical diagnosis and should not be used in this way.

Intellectual testing These tests comprise notably the Weschler Adult Intelligence Scale (WAIS) together with some accessory tests of verbal (e.g. the Mill Hill Vocabulary Scale) and non-verbal (e.g. Raven's Progressive Matrices) ability, which correlate closely with IQ. Their routine clinical application in functional illnesses is uncommon; occasionally, the finding of low or borderline subnormal intelligence makes unexpected sense of an unclear clinical picture.

Miscellaneous psychological tests A bewildering array of psychological investigations, all of a more or less recondite nature, have been devised, and sometimes crop up in psychologists' reports. While the results of such tests might throw light on individual cases, by and large they have no diagnostic significance. Examples range from the Rorschach test, which has been shown to have little intrinsic validity, to procedures like the Repertory Grid and sorting tasks; these almost certainly reveal important psychological deficits in psychosis, but their exact status remains uncertain.

Nursing observations

The patient's weight may be an important diagnostic and prognostic pointer in depressive disorders and some organic disorders. Weekly weighing is also valuable as a measure of progress, e.g. in recovery from a depressive illness. Also in depressive disorders a valuable investigation is the detailed recording of the patient's sleep pattern. Nurses may also complete some rating scales (see above).

Organic disorders: the acute confusional state

Physical investigations

Except when the cause of an acute confusional state is self-evident (as in some toxic delirious states or following head injury) or can be easily pinpointed (for instance, urinary tract infection in an elderly woman), the routine physical investigations described above for functionally ill patients form a useful starting point for physical investigation of the confused patient. These can then be supplemented with further investigations suggested by the nature of the presentation, such as urine bacteriology or more detailed blood biochemistry. A lengthy series of physical investigations with no definite indication, should, however, never be embarked upon. There should at the very least be consultation with senior members of the psychiatric team and preferably referral to a physician. The trainee who orders EEGs, CAT scans and intravenous pyelograms indiscriminately will soon antagonize senior members of his own and other disciplines.

Psychological investigations

In general these have no part to play in the diagnosis of an acute confusional state. The taking of a good cognitive state examination (see Chapter 6) is all that is required. If desired, this can be supplemented by a more extensive evaluation such as that described by Withers and Hinton.

Organic disorders: dementia

Physical investigations

The goal of physical investigations in a clinically obvious dementing illness is to rule out any treatable cause; a lesser aim is to specify the nature of the disease process more precisely; finally there may be a need in younger patients to confirm the diagnosis by objective physical tests, so as to spare relatives further false hope.

The first step is physical examination which should include a full neurological assessment and, often forgotten, a search for vascular disease (see Chapter 7). Next, the routine physical investigations described earlier may be carried out, as these cover most of the treatable possibilities for dementia. Thyroid function tests should also be performed; very occasionally, hypothyroidism may present with cognitive impairment in the absence of any other stigmata of the disease. An ECG should be obtained as part of the assessment of cardiovascular status.

Further investigations are often undertaken, but should not be considered routine. The EEG may remain normal in a clinically well-advanced dementia; likewise CT scan changes of cerebral atrophy correlate only poorly with clinical status. Factors that incline the psychiatrist to a more extensive investigation include presentation in the presenium, as mentioned above, and also an atypical clinical picture. Dementias with an unusual mode of onset or with peculiar features sometimes betray a treatable cause: an example is normal pressure hydrocephalus with its clinical triad of fluctuating cognitive impairment, apraxic gait disturbance and incontinence; if confirmed by CAT scan appearance and dynamic studies, this condition may respond favourably to a CSF shunting procedure.

Psychological investigations

In the presence of clinically obvious cognitive deficits, detailed tests of intellectual functioning such as the WAIS can contribute no new information and are irrelevant. In a few instances, the pattern of deficits on intellectual testing may point to a particular diagnostic category of dementia; very rarely a striking variability in test results with preservation of some, but not other, abilities might raise the possibility that the illness is, in reality a depressive pseudo-dementia.

Alcohol and drug intoxication

Patients with uncomplicated alcohol or drug intoxication are unlikely to be referred initially to psychiatric services, but since clinical pictures resembling intoxication may be caused by other conditions such as, for example, head injury, lobar pneumonia, and hypoglycaemia, patients who appear to be intoxicated with alcohol or drugs on referral require careful physical examination and investigation before psychiatric admission. Breath alcohol analysis and urine toxicological screening may yield results which contradict the clinical diagnosis of intoxication. Examination may reveal a coexistent medical or traumatic disorder which requires medical or surgical intervention. Serial monitoring of conscious level with the *Glasgow Coma Scale* may point to a deteriorating or unexpectedly slowly recovering conscious level in the patient who is being 'detoxified'.

FURTHER INVESTIGATION OF THE PSYCHIATRIC PATIENT

Psychiatry abounds with patients in whom organic disorders present functionally, in whom there is simultaneous psychiatric and physical disease, and a few, in the evolution of whose disorders, functional and organic factors are inextricably intertwined. Such cases are among the most interesting, challenging and sometimes the most rewarding to investigate and treat.

The key to investigation of such patients is the taking of a coherent and detailed psychiatric history. This necessitates the often tedious business of obtaining information from informants, reading the patient's general practice file, sending for previous hospital records, and assembling all the information into chronological order. However, at the very least, this approach saves unnecessary repetition of investigations and quite often it narrows the range of diagnostic possibilities considerably. All too commonly, patients are seen who have been examined at length by psychiatrists, neurologists and physicians, referred to specialist units, subjected to a spectacular range of investigations, all to no avail; yet, as soon as the trainee troubles to take the history from an informant and chart the course of the illness from the beginning, the diagnosis, never really that obscure, becomes obvious.

This section provides some guidelines for the further investigation of psychiatric patients whose status as functional, for one reason or another, becomes questioned. Somewhat arbitrarily, these cases can be divided into *the suspected symptomatic illness, the suspected confusional state, and the suspected early dementia.*

The suspected symptomatic illness

As described above, some physical diseases have the potential to produce psychiatric complications that are not accompanied by confusion and which do not occur in the setting of global intellectual deterioration. Such quasi-functional states are usually referred to as *symptomatic* or *secondary* and it is presumed that the physical disorder has, in some way, released a specific psychopathological process.

Apparently functional mental states tend to become suspected of being symptomatic in various contexts. An atypical clinical picture should always raise this possibility, though such presentations are almost commonplace in psychiatry and many become more typical with the passage of time. The finding of abnormal results on routine physical investigation should likewise institute a systematic search for an organic causal basis to the psychiatric disorder. Finally, patients with known chronic physical ailments who develop psychiatric symptoms are good candidates for having a symptomatic psychiatric state. This statement may seem obvious, but not infrequently the possibility is overlooked, or the co-existence of conditions arbitrarily dismissed as coincidence. Diseases with a high risk of symptomatic psychiatric complications include epilepsy, connective tissue and endocrine disorders.

Excessive drinking, alcohol dependence and drug abuse, which may be covert, can cause quasi-functional psychiatric complications which range from non-specific pictures to florid psychotic states. Blood, breath and urine analyses, performed at random, are thus always worthwhile in any patient whose symptoms are suspect in any way whatsoever. In one case, it was only after innumerable admissions and finally leucotomy, that a cache of amphetamines was discovered in the patient's locker!

The suspected confusional state

Sometimes, patients present with a psychotic picture whose abrupt onset, fluctuating course and presence of visual hallucinations for instance, suggest they may be suffering from an acute confusional state. Objective signs of confusion, however, in the sense of routine cognitive state abnormalities, are not demonstrable. Confusional states can be subtle, and their detection is of the utmost importance, not only for the purposes of treatment but also to prevent the wrongful acquisition of a label of psychosis, with all the social and occupational stigmatization this entails.

An important first step is to obtain an independent history from an informant; this may reveal strong suggestions of organicity (e.g. confusion at night prior to admission), or alternatively might point to an unsuspected toxic factor (such as alcohol or drug abuse). Repeated, detailed cognitive state examinations are the other principal means of establishing the diagnosis. Acute confusional states characteristically fluctuate, and so clouding of consciousness that is absent at one point may become evident later, for instance at the end of the day when the patient is tired. Similarly, recall may appear intact during one examination, but the next day the patient has no recollection of having been examined the day before. Other clinical clues to an illness being confusional in nature include a tendency to lose the thread of demanding conversation, slowness of mentation, fatiguability, and restless sleep accompanied by vivid dreams. These factors are discussed more fully by Mayer Gross, Slater and Roth.

Physical investigations can provide important corroborative evidence for the presence of underlying organic disease. Basic temperature and pulse monitoring, often neglected on psychiatric wards, may point to occult infection; the white cell count and ESR and plasma viscosity (PV) can also be indicative of this and should be repeated at intervals. Another useful procedure is EEG examination: this tends to show non-specific slowing in confusional states of any cause. While not in itself diagnostic, if the EEG improves on recovery, the diagnosis is confirmed. Rarely, in confused patients with no prior history of epilepsy the EEG will show the marked paroxysmal abnormalities of epileptic status.

Psychological testing has little part to play in the investigation of a subtle confusional state. In some instances, an extended cognitive state evaluation (like that of Withers and Hinton) may reveal deficits not amounting to disorientation, but which go beyond those attributable to a functional psychiatric state. Repeated testing might show a variation in test scores paralleling the fluctuation in conscious level.

The suspected early dementia

In their early stages, dementing illnesses can be complicated by psychiatric symptoms of many different types. If the intellectual deterioration is minor and the psychiatric symptomatology pronounced, the patient is liable to be diagnosed as suffering from a functional illness, this only being revised months, or even years, later. Among elderly patients in particular, a differential diagnosis of early dementia almost always has to be considered.

Once again, it is the obtaining of a detailed history from an informant that is often the key to establishing the diagnosis. Relatives may have to be probed, even asked leading questions, but will then go on to provide a wealth of information about personality changes, errors of judgement, narrowing interests, deterioration in personal habits and so on, all pointing to insidious organic deterioration. Physical examination can add important circumstantial evidence to this; there may be signs of widespread vascular disease, or neurological findings, equivocal or unequivocal might be present.

Physical investigations, beyond those already detailed as routine, are usually unhelpful. The EEG is commonly normal and, if not, tends to show only non-specific, minor abnormalities. It is, however, worth performing since if repeated a few months later it may show progressive deterioration. CAT scanning is subject to difficulties of interpretation: appearances indicating cerebral atrophy are common in the middle-aged to elderly population, but the significance of this is currently uncertain.

It is, however, psychological investigations that can yield the greatest rewards in investigation of a suspected early dementia. While routine cognitive state examination may reveal no abnormalities, more extended evaluation using the Withers and Hinton tests can often reveal gaps in knowledge and deficient abilities which are highly suggestive of organic deterioration. Formal intellectual testing may add decisive evidence. The patient's overall intelligence quotient (IQ) is not usually reduced to a degree out of keeping with background and attainments; there may, however, be a discrepancy between verbal and performance IQ scores, or between tested IQ and that expected on the basis of reading ability. Other signs, notably a marked scatter of sub-test scores or disparity between memory and intelligence quotients, have also been held to be important indices of organic intellectual decline.

CONCLUSION

It should be added that what may be considered investigation in psychiatry goes far beyond the formal physical and psychological tests detailed in this chapter. This is particularly true in functional disorders, where diagnosis still depends primarily on clinical judgement. Here, the systematic collection of information from as many sources as possible is all important as the only means of substantiation of a particular view. Investigation of these patients should always include careful analysis of family history, social background and pre-morbid personality as described, for example, in *Fish's Clinical Psychopathology.* Even in straightforward cases, this can radically affect a formulation. In patients with long, complicated or obscure histories, it can make all the difference. Inquiry into a family history need not stop at questioning of the patient; relatives' hospital records can be obtained. Information about social circumstances is relatively easily obtained from social work or probation reports, but this sometimes lacks the dramatic impact of a home visit by the trainee. Psychiatric illnesses are always coloured, and sometimes grossly distorted by, the patients' pre-morbid personality. If such investigation is cursory and does not extend to independent confirmation from an informant, erroneous impressions are gained with occasionally disastrous consequences for management. Such 'social' investigations can sometimes make the diagnosis, uncover a simplifying explanation, or even reveal that a string of diagnoses which are nothing more than labels has been acquired. The weighing and sifting of clinical and social information, rather than formal physical and psychological tests, remains, perhaps, the most important aspect of investigation in psychiatry.

Further reading

Brierley CE, Szabadi E, Rix KJB and Bradshaw CM (in preparation) The Manchester nurse rating scales for the daily simultaneous assessment of depressive and manic ward behaviours

Hamilton M (1978) *Fish's Outline of Psychiatry, 3rd edition.* Bristol: John Wright and Sons

Mayer Gross W, Slater E and Roth M (1969) *Clinical Psychiatry, 3rd edition.* London: Baillière Tindall and Cassell

Montgomery SA and Åsberg M (1979) A new depression rating scale designed to be sensitive to change. *British Journal of Psychiatry 134:* 382–389

Rix KJB and Lumsden Rix EM (1983) Alcohol intoxication. In *Alcohol Problems,* pp.32–47. Bristol: Wright, PSG

Withers E and Hinton J (1979) Three forms of the clinical tests of the sensorium and their reliability. *British Journal of Psychiatry 119:* 1–8

Zigmond AS and Snaith RP (1983) The Hospital Anxiety and Depression Scale. *Acta Psychiatrica Scandinavica 67:* 361–370

9

The Formulation

Digby Tantam & Maurice Greenberg

There are a number of reasons why the understanding and management of psychiatric patients appear complicated: the diagnosis may be uncertain, the relative importance of particular events to the development of the disorder may be unclear, and doubt may exist about the efficacy of alternative treatments. Even on those rare occasions when the answers to these questions appear to be clear-cut, management may still prove difficult because too little attention has been paid to the patient as an individual, and how he or she might respond.

The formulation* provides a framework for selecting and organizing information which takes these uncertainties into consideration, and enables the individual aspects of a particular patient to be incorporated. It is a discursive account organized under the following five headings:

1. Summary (descriptive formulation)
2. Differential diagnosis
3. Aetiology
4. Management
5. Prognosis

A useful formulation will illuminate why a particular patient has developed a particular disorder at a particular time. It will also guide the management in a direction that is most useful for that patient.

Following this approach from the first contact with the patient enables the psychiatrist to organize his thoughts in a logical fashion while at the same time retaining the individual, narrative quality, that brings the patient to life.

---

*MRCPsych examination candidates should note that the College refers to the 'formulation' as the 'assessment'.

An essential component of a psychiatrist's management skills is the ability to communicate effectively with people who have a wide range of psychiatric knowledge, and who require information for a variety of reasons. The framework provided by the formulation helps so long as three basic constraints are recognized: (1) the person with whom one is communicating, (2) the reason why the information is needed, and (3) the amount of time available for communication. For example, when the trainee has examined a potentially suicidal patient in the casualty department and has decided that he may need to admit this patient formally to the ward, he will need to communicate this to the patient, the patient's relatives, the ward sister, a social worker and, often, a senior colleague. Each communication will be based upon the same information, but will be modified by the above factors. Each will involve a formulation but its detail and emphasis will probably differ for each recipient.

In this chapter it is assumed that the information is being presented to a consultant in a ward-round, and that there are no time constraints beyond those that normally apply to this situation. Once the trainee has developed the general principles which can only be acquired through clinical practice, they can be readily applied to formulations suitable for any other situation, including the MRCPsych clinical examinations.

FACTS AND INFERENCE

It is always safe to assume that no single inference will go unchallenged and that it is essential to be able to justify any one that is made. The formulation is itself a kind of argument, starting out as a critical review of the evidence, and then taking into account knowledge of other cases and other related situations to build up a recommendation for a particular course of action. Valid clinical judgements are unlikely to be reached from inaccurate facts, and it is therefore important to establish their accuracy before proceeding to any deductions about diagnosis, aetiology, management or prognosis. Judgements about the meaning or importance of the facts should be deferred to these later sections.

A major source of weakness in formulations is a failure to distinguish between fact and inference. A typical example of this is when a patient is described as presenting with 'third person auditory hallucinations', whereas he really presented with the complaint that "I heard two people talking about me, saying that I wasn't to be trusted". The latter is a 'fact', whereas the former is a psychiatric 'inference', based upon other information such as whether the patient was alone at the time, or whether he was convinced that the experience was real and not imagined.

Accurate reporting of what is said by the patient, or informant, helps clarify the distinction between fact and inference. This not only facilitates a useful dialogue about why the psychiatrist has arrived at particular conclusions, it also helps bring the patient alive in the presentation.

SUMMARY

It is only necessary to introduce such facts as are relevant to the subsequent formulation. The descriptive formulation will not be a summary of the full psychiatric history and examination, but a selective extract, mainly from the history of the presenting illness and the mental state examination. But in some patients important facts about the family history, about the physical examination or, indeed, about any of the areas covered in the full interview might be relevant.

The account of the present illness needs to be both brief, and reasonably simple, in order to focus attention effectively. Aim for a length of one or two paragraphs and try to keep facts in a strict chronological sequence, starting either with the previous treatment of a similar illness, or with the onset of the present illness and the surrounding circumstances.

There should always be a statement of any factors that have been associated with a worsening or an improvement of the symptoms, and there should always be some statement about the patient's principal symptoms. The descriptive formulation should conclude with an account of how much the patient is presently affected by the symptoms, and an account of the present mental state.

It makes for duplication to include mental state information in the history, and past information should obviously not be included in the current mental state, since what is needed is an assessment of the patient now. Imagine that you have to transfer the patient to a medical ward as an emergency: you would want to tell the medical staff there about the patient's present psychiatric condition, not how he got into that condition. However, it would not be wise to restrict your assessment of the patient's condition to your interview with the patient. The fluctuations in mental state, the effect of a different social situation and the wish of some patients to conceal abnormalities make the patient's apparent mental state during the interview only a guide to their state of mind. It is therefore usual to incorporate reports of experiences or behaviour occurring in the period immediately preceding the examination. For example, if a tense, obviously distracted man, who has been acutely disturbed for a week, denied auditory hallucinations on examination, it would be appropriate to include in the account of his mental state the fact that, when he was admitted, he had alluded to accusing voices.

Occasionally information about past mental state assessments is available. This is best inserted into the history of the present illness, prefaced with some introductory statement like "Her mental state at that time was reported as . . ".

One purpose of the mental state examination is to check normal psychological functioning, but the fact that phobic Mr X has no evidence of cognitive failure or that obsessional Miss Y is not deluded may have little bearing on their diagnosis or management. Only those findings which are relevant should be included in the summary. Abnormalities are almost always relevant, as is a brief account of appearance and insight. Negative findings need not be repeated unless they serve to disconfirm some diagnostic or aetiological hypothesis.

Avoid technical terms as much as possible. Give brief, factual descriptions of the phenomena. Do not say, for example, that Mrs Z is auditorily hallucinated, but say that she hears the voice of her long-deceased mother giving her instructions. Disagreements about what the patient has experienced will then be resolved before differences of opinion about what these experiences might indicate are discussed.

DIFFERENTIAL DIAGNOSIS

This may start with a statement about the confidence with which a diagnosis can be made. In some cases, for example, you may be dubious even whether the patient is ill at all and will want to discuss this before considering diagnosis. In other cases the diagnosis may be very clear-cut and you may want to mention alternative diagnoses simply to dismiss them.

Try not to consider more than three or four diagnoses seriously and try to narrow the field down as much as possible to one corner of ICD-9. Diagnostic terms should be drawn from its Glossary, although other terms, for example, from DSM-III, can sometimes be justified, but will need explanation. Give a succinct account of the reasons why some diagnoses may be applicable and why the preferred diagnosis is the most likely of these.

Sometimes a single diagnosis is not adequate and supplementary diagnoses have to be made. Common supplementary diagnoses are epilepsy, alcohol or drug abuse/dependence and personality disorder. Remember that any supplementary diagnosis also needs justification. A supplementary diagnosis should be made only if the condition diagnosed is independent of the main diagnosis. For example, it is not justifiable to make a supplementary diagnosis of 'obsessional personality disorder' in a man with methodical habits who had no symptoms until he developed an obsessional neurosis, nor is a supplementary diagnosis of 'alcohol abuse' warranted in a woman who drinks heavily when she is depressed but otherwise has a normal pattern of drinking. This is not to say that these factors are not important. They are. The woman's use of alcohol may very well need consideration when management is discussed, and the man's personality should be considered with other potential aetiological factors.

AETIOLOGY

Many psychiatrists aspire to be eclectic, but very few succeed. There is a bias towards one or other kind of aetiological explanation. Aetiological speculation often seems to be a source of embarrassment and is almost always the skimpiest part of some formulations. It may be that trainees realise how unlikely it is for a complete explanation to be given of why the patient became ill, and why his or her illness took the form that it did. However, by careful reasoning about the timing and about the associations between different events, it is often possible to go surprisingly far towards preparing the ground for management, by identifying underlying causes. One does not need a deep understanding of family dynamics to be able to conclude, for example, that family influence was not a significant factor in the breakdown of a patient with schizophrenia when his hospital admissions were rather more frequent when he was living alone in a boarding house than when he was living with his family.

The best approach is to consider every possible aetiological hypothesis systematically. Thus it may be necessary to have a mental checklist of the different kinds of aetiological explanation used in psychiatry. It is always worth considering the following three factors:

- physical – for example, genetic factors, constitutional factors, and factors relating to recent bodily derangement due to physical illness or drug intoxication;
- social/cultural – for example, income, employment, housing, culture, and other indicators of special status, advantage, and integration;
- personal – for example, personality, and the quality and availability of current social relationships.

Information about personality is often of particular importance, but it may sometimes be difficult to obtain directly. Patients and their relatives are often unwilling to be analytic or to seem critical when asked to assess personality, and may give rather bland answers to direct questions. Some information will have to be obtained by inference from the personal history, noting the way that the patient has surmounted difficulties, and the strength and durability of relationships (for further details of personality examination see pp.68–71).

Within each of the three aetiological categories, it is often worth distinguishing between remote events, which are likely to include those factors which predisposed to the illness ('predisposing factors') and more recent circumstances and events which may have caused a period of vulnerability ('vulnerability factors') or precipitated the illness ('provoking factors'). Pathoplastic factors, which influence the way in which the psychiatric disorder presents itself, may be either remote or recent. For example, the fact that a very turbulent adolescent with a deprived upbringing has turned to alcohol may be partly attributed to the remote pathoplastic effect of his father's characteristic behaviour. The fact that he has a tendency to present to hospital with abdominal pain subsequently found to have no organic aetiology, is more likely to be due to the pathoplastic effect of the hospital admission for appendicitis that occurred recently.

MANAGEMENT

The formulation of the diagnosis or aetiological hypothesis will often throw into relief inconsistencies in the information available or uncertainty about the conclusions to be drawn from it. The first step in management is, therefore, to consider further investigations (see Chapter 8).

Further investigations

When formulating a case, investigations should be presented in order to test the current diagnostic or aetiological hypotheses, and screening investigations should therefore be omitted, unless they can be justified in these terms. It may be helpful to categorize investigations under the headings described above: physical, social/cultural and personal. However, it makes clinical sense to present them in the order that they would be most efficiently carried out, which is usually in ascending order of cost and invasiveness.

Obtaining further information from an informant will therefore often be one of the first investigations to be considered. It is important to be specific about who it should be, what information is required, and which particular hypothesis it is intended to test.

The informant will often be the patient's nearest relative, but it may be a general practitioner, an employer, a school teacher, or another psychiatrist who has previously treated the patient. Specifying the purpose of the enquiry has practical implications, and is necessary, whatever the investigation. One frequent investigation is 'to obtain the old notes'. However, it is not uncommon for the old records to be obtained, studied, and sent back, without being used to answer important questions about the patient, usually because the questions have not been formulated.

Often the next step in investigation will be assessment by other members of the team. It is quite unhelpful clinically, and inadequate in a formulation, to recommend 'psychometry' or 'ward observation' as an investigation. These instructions are equivalent to asking that the patient be 'X-rayed'. The purpose of the investigation, the area to be investigated and, if possible, the type of investigation to be carried out should be clearly specified.

The same principle applies to physical investigations. In every case the specific test, or group of tests, and the reason for each should be stated.

Treatment

It is tempting at this stage, after so much reasoned discussion, to simply state a recommended treatment, such as 'antidepressants' or 'psychotherapy', and to move on. In clinical practice, it is not so easy. Patients do not always agree with our assessments, and sometimes refuse treatment, or make recommendations of their own. It may, for example, be a less difficult clinical decision that an antidepressant should be given to a particular patient than the decision about where it should be given, and by whom. The formulation should reflect these clinical realities.

It often clarifies a formulation of the treatment to consider the treatment of the episode of illness separately from longer term treatment, and it may again be useful to make use of the physical, social/cultural and personal categories. However, consideration of the treatment of the current episode should start with the basics: 1) whether any treatment is indicated; 2) who will be concerned with the treatment and what they should be told; 3) whether it should be carried out on an out-, day- or in-patient basis; and, 4) if the patient requires admission, whether this will need to be on a formal or an informal basis.

If there is a definitive treatment for the condition, this should be discussed first, in a practical manner and taking account of the patient's circumstances. For example, it is not sufficient to say of a woman with agoraphobia, that "I would treat her behaviourally" or of a man with schizophrenia, "Antipsychotic drug treatment is indicated". Your treatment plan should describe accurately what you would do in practice, and the reasons why you have chosen a particular course of action. For example, "This woman is firmly convinced that she is ill and has rejected psychological treatment in the past because she thinks it inappropriate. Therefore the origin of her physical symptoms in anxiety should be explained, and the role of learning and anticipation in anxiety generation discussed. It would be useful to involve the patient's husband in these discussions, because there is a suggestion that he could be reinforcing her symptoms. When this has been done, it is probably best that she is referred to a clinical psychologist for a more detailed behavioural assessment and design of a treatment programme. This can then be carried out under the supervision of a nurse on the ward and with the assistance of her husband".

A discussion of drug treatment should begin with the choice of drug. This will depend upon the secondary effects of the drug, such as the amount of sedation it induces. It will also depend upon the possible unwanted effects, and what can be done about them; and on availability of a particular preparation, for example the use of a mixture in the case of a patient who may not swallow a tablet. This section should also include the starting dose, the indications for increasing the dose, the rate and level of increase, and most important, a statement about the length of treatment, which should include some consideration of what would prompt a reconsideration of the treatment strategy.

The precision with which the type, frequency, administration and justification of treatment is specified is particularly important in the case of dynamic psychotherapy. To say that "This patient needs psychotherapy" is about as helpful as saying "This patient needs drugs" or "The patient should be observed".

It should always be assumed that treatment will be discussed fully with the patient. Usually this will result in patients accepting reasonable treatment, and the question of consent will not need to be discussed in the formulation. However, it may sometimes be necessary to consider whether treatment should be given without the patient's consent. For example, a depressed patient with nihilistic delusions may benefit most from ECT, but may be quite likely to refuse it on the grounds that no treatment will work, or that it will only make him worse. In such a case the indications and procedure for compulsory treatment should be considered.

Treatment which is supplementary to the definitive treatment given for the patient's main condition will often need to be discussed. For example, the depressed patient receiving an antidepressant may also benefit from cognitive therapy, and the acutely schizophrenic patient may need a sedative antipsychotic given at night as a hypnotic. It is worth remembering that psychological and social factors are frequently important, even in conditions which have a physical basis. Contrarily, drug treatment may well be indicated occasionally for the temporary relief of psychogenic disturbance.

Common symptoms or problems which may call for supplementary treatment include insomnia, acute anxiety, psychotic episodes, suicidal thoughts, aggression, and any physical disorder from which the patient may be suffering.

Longer-term treatment

Many psychiatric disorders have a tendency to recur. They may also leave some degree of disability which may be as much due to the associated stigma as to the disorder itself. The prevention of relapse and the reduction of disability are therefore important features of the management of many patients.

In this discussion, as elsewhere, it is essential to be practical and to stick closely to the needs of the individual patient. This is best achieved by mentally reviewing a comprehensive list of sub-headings and selecting those that are relevant for discussion.

Reduction of relapse

Maintenance treatment will usually need to be considered in a case of affective disorder or schizophrenia. Long-term treatment may also need to be considered in other disorders such as alcohol dependence in which the use of disulfiram may be indicated. However, it is worth remembering that the benefits of maintenance treatment are usually much less obvious than those of acute treatment, and the costs often higher. It will therefore need careful formulation, particularly as patients are much less likely to comply with maintenance treatment if they cannot be convinced of its value.

The avoidance or reduction of provoking factors will include a wide range of measures, from family therapy in the case of a schizophrenic patient's emotionally demanding household, to the avoidance of marijuana, when this has been shown to trigger relapse. Since it is impossible to change everything that may be harmful to the patient, it is best to be realistic and to emphasize those factors which appear most important, and are also most likely to be changeable.

It may not seem to be realistic to reduce vulnerability in the case of a frequently relapsing disorder. However, even in hereditary disorders the effects of the disorder can be ameliorated by protective factors. Some of these can be altered. Self-esteem can be increased by the provision of satisfaction and support through appropriate work or occupation and through social relationships. New coping mechanisms can be taught which cushion the effects of adversity or worry, or which are more effective in combating a mild recurrence of symptoms before serious relapse can occur. The formulation of the management will usually require some mention of these or other protective factors. It is this part of the formulation which is likely to be of greatest interest to the patient and the concerned relative.

Reduction of disability

Alternative ways of reducing disability will need to be

considered in the management of most patients with schizophrenia, in other psychotic patients, and in patients with a chronic neurosis, such as obsessional disorder. It is in this section that rehabilitation should be considered. Rehabilitation may involve learning new skills relevant to independent life, such as literacy, and these skills may be very mundane, e.g. learning to cook or to collect a disability pension. Rehabilitation begins immediately that the patient is admitted into hospital, with the steps that are taken to prevent the patient from losing independence unnecessarily.

PROGNOSIS

One of the commonest questions that the relatives ask of a newly admitted patient with a first episode of illness is "Will they get better?". The formulation of the prognosis is therefore a skill that junior psychiatrists put to regular practical use. The prognosis is also the yardstick by which treatment must be evaluated. It is best to start the formulation of the prognosis with the basics: whether the patient's present condition will change and if so, when, and will it be for the worse or the better.

Once the short-term prognosis has been considered, then the long-term can be discussed and this will usually mean commenting on the persistence of symptoms, the likelihood of relapse and the patient's future capacity to lead a normal, i.e. successful and responsible, life. The prognosis for each of these may be different; for example, it is possible for patients to continue experiencing auditory hallucinations and at the same time to have successfully returned to their work and family.

The former, *symptomatic*, prognosis may be of particular interest to another doctor, but the latter, *social*, prognosis is likely to be of more interest to the family. The prognosis is, like the rest of the formulation, aimed at someone, and its content will be influenced by the questions that this person wants answered. Sometimes these may be very specific: is a sick doctor likely to be able to return to work, for example?

Often such questions cannot be answered, partly because the course of the disorder will be influenced by future events. These may sometimes need to be considered in the prognosis as, for example, in the case of a first episode of psychosis occurring in the puerperium. The prognosis for no recurrence is good if the woman does not become pregnant again, but there is a significant chance of relapse if she does.

Treatment and compliance with treatment are other factors which will usually affect prognosis, and it is often useful to consider the outcome of the untreated disorder as well as the outcome that the patient can expect if treatment is followed.

It is correct to be qualified in a prognosis, and wrong to be over-precise. On the other hand, it is important to strive to be as precise as possible. The comments 'good' or 'guarded' are insufficient by themselves, since they do not specify either the factors which would improve prognosis, or in what respects the prognosis is either good or bad.

CONCLUDING REMARKS

Formulating the management and prognosis of psychiatric cases, like reviewing a research paper or summing-up from the Bench, requires a format which has to be learnt, a conscious review of all the facts and the possible disputes which may arise from them, and practice in blending abstract knowledge with individual facts in such a way as to get the most practical utility out of them.

The practice cannot be circumvented, and is undeniably tedious because great pains may not be crowned with success, at least in the early stages. However, we hope that we have been able to convey something of the intellectual interest of formulating psychiatric cases, an interest which we think derives from the fusion of practical knowledge of humanity with the anonymous findings of medical science and which, for us, is one of the appeals of psychiatry.

A SPECIMEN FORMULATION

Summary

Mrs. A. is a 47-year-old housewife who is separated and has been temporarily living with her sister. She was transferred from the medical ward where she had been admitted with chest pain. She was very distressed at the time of the transfer and said "I want to leave my body. I've never been so out of control in my life".

She describes herself as being "a worrier" for years, and has had treatment for tension-related headaches in the past, especially over the last seven years. Six months ago Mrs. A. became acutely ill with chest pain and was admitted to a medical ward in a Bristol hospital. She says that she was told that she had an inflammation of the heart, but after three days she was transferred to a psychiatric unit. A summary from the hospital states that all investigations were normal and that she was noted to be extremely anxious.

At the time of that admission, Mrs. A. was living in a hostel. On discharge she decided to move from Bristol to London to be nearer her family. She initially stayed with her brother, but they got on badly and for the two weeks before admission Mrs. A. had been living with a sister. Her chest pain returned three weeks ago, and for the two weeks before admission she was taking large doses of diazepam from a stock which her sister had. She denied drinking alcohol regularly, or to excess.

On direct questioning, Mrs. A. admits that if she thinks about her family's rejection of her or she dwells too much on her future, she "gets so worked up" that she can hardly breathe. On these occasions, she also experiences tingling in her fingers, headaches, sweating, and a churning in her stomach. She estimates that she has lost about 2 lb. in weight in the last six months. She says that her sleep and her mood were almost back to normal at the time that she moved to London, but that she has been feeling more tense and having trouble getting to sleep since she started rowing with her brother. She felt very unhappy when he asked her to move, but was not previously low. Her concentration was poor and she did not want to pursue her normal interests.

Mrs. A. has had one previous episode of psychiatric treatment, 15 years ago, when she was in hospital for three weeks and was treated with antidepressants. Her family and personal history is also relevant. A brother and her father both died of complications of alcoholism. She has three surviving older brothers and two younger sisters, but has no close relationship with them. Her mother, from whom she is estranged, has diabetes and has recently had a heart attack.

She was born in Trinidad but came to this country with her parents when she was two. She was, she says, the "black sheep of the family" and described her life as very unhappy, especially after her father left her mother when she was seven after a good deal of family violence. Her mother subsequently lived with a man whom she described as "a bastard" but refused to say why. Her only confidant within the family was her mother's mother who died seven years ago.

Mrs. A. became pregnant at the age of 15. She had the child, but split up with the father and supported herself by prostitution. In her early 20s she became involved with an older woman and lived with her for 10 years. The break-up of this relationship precipitated her first hospital admission. For 15 years she has had regular work as a care assistant, either wih the elderly or with disturbed adolescents. She married a younger man four years before admission, but the relationship was never good, and he left her after a year. She has only the one child, the son, who is now 31 and with whom she keeps in distant contact.

On examination she was wearing sloppy, casually put on clothes. She looked older than her years, smoked heavily during the interview, and moved restlessly in her chair. Her speech was rapid, and her voice and face animated. She asked several times for reassurance about her heart, and cried when talking about her brother's recent behaviour and when talking about her childhood. She said that she was feeling "awful". She appeared tense, but not sad. She worried about the future, but did not feel hopeless and had never thought of suicide. There was no evidence that Mrs. A. had abnormal experiences or beliefs, and her cognition was unimpaired.

She had a blood pressure of 160/100 but physical examination was otherwise normal.

Differential diagnosis

Mrs. A. has suffered a relapse of a non-psychotic illness which began six months before admission. The differential diagnosis lies between a depressive illness or an anxiety-related illness. Depression is a common complication of anxiety-related disorders, and may co-exist with them, but Mrs. A. does not in fact have many symptoms of depression. She is anxious rather than low, and she has not lost much weight, is not waking early in the morning, and is not hopeless about the future. She does have many anxiety symptoms, however, and an anxiety-related disorder is most likely.

Although Mrs. A's anxiety waxes and wanes, exacerbations are triggered by ruminations rather than situations. A diagnosis of agoraphobia (DSM-III panic disorder) is not therefore appropriate, and the most likely diagnosis is:

A. anxiety state (ICD 300.0) (DSM-III 300.02 generalized anxiety disorder).

Mrs. A. has the capacity to make a long-term intimate relationship, and has apparently been able to hold an emotionally demanding job. There are no grounds for making a diagnosis of a personality disorder. Her excessive use of diazepam before admission may indicate a long-term abuse of non-prescribed tranquillizers. There is no evidence from the history that Mrs. A. has suffered social or health consequences even if she has been taking drugs, but closer scrutiny may reveal these. A possible supplementary diagnosis should therefore be considered:

B. ?non-dependent abuse of tranquillizers (ICD 305.4) (DSM-III sedative abuse).

Mrs. A's chest pain is clearly related to anxiety, and she has had it previously investigated, and there is no evidence of cardiovascular disease on physical examination. Chest pain may be produced by hyperventilation, and is a common symptom of anxiety. However a physical cause of chest pain should be ruled out.

Thyrotoxicosis should always be considered as a cause of anxiety. Mrs. A. has no signs of thyrotoxicosis and has not lost weight, however. The much rarer condition of phaeochromocytoma may be associated with episodic anxiety, usually associated with flushing and headache. About half the patients with this tumour have hypertension. It is not, however, associated with persistent anxiety.

The two most likely physical conditions are:

C. 1. ??myocardial ischaemia
or 2. ??mitral valve prolapse
but 3. ??thyrotoxicosis needs to be considered.

Aetiology

Parental discord in childhood predisposes to later anxiety disorder in women. There is also evidence of a common hereditary risk for both alcoholism and mood disorder. Mrs. A. is thus predisposed to anxiety both psychologically and possibly also genetically.

Mrs. A's difficulties in making close relationships with men may point to a sexual problem. Her characterization of her step-father as a bastard may point to sexual harassment or incest. If incest has occurred, this may make her work with disturbed adolescents simultaneously fascinating and stressful, and may have contributed to her anxiety.

Mrs. A's anxiety seems to have worsened after her grandmother's death. This grandmother was the family member closest to Mrs. A. in childhood, and it is possible that Mrs. A's mourning was never completed. Unresolved grief may be one cause of chronic anxiety or anxiety-proneness, and so this may be another vulnerability factor.

The precipitant of Mrs. A's anxiety attack six months before admission is unknown. It is possible that there was a physical cause, but that the symptoms were maintained by psychological factors, possibly related to Mrs. A's feelings about her mother's heart disease. The most recent episode was clearly related to the deterioration in her relationship with her brother. She put it clearly when she said, "Now I've lost everyone".

Management

There are a number of loose threads in Mrs. A's case that need to be tied in. Further history from Mrs. A. will throw light on whether there was incest in her childhood, and what effect this has had. More details about Mrs. A's response to her grandmother's death are also needed. The sister could confirm some details of the history, may be able to contribute an assessment of Mrs. A's personality, and may be able to give more details about Mrs. A's drug taking.

It would be useful to obtain the records of Mrs. A's physical illness, and of her previous psychiatric treatment.

Obtaining a urine sample for drug analysis and blood for routine biochemistry and thyroid function studies, having her chest X-rayed, and looking at an ECG are the most important special investigations to perform immediately.

Whether or not Mrs. A. should be admitted to hospital will depend on the extent and chronicity of her distress, and the level of support and tolerance from her sister. The investigations and the treatment could equally well be carried out as an in- or an out-patient.

The immediate goal in the treatment of anxiety is to restore Mrs. A's sense of self-control by reducing the severity of her symptoms, by helping her to understand them as psychological manifestations, and by teaching her techniques to control, prevent or anticipate them. Mrs. A's anxiety symptoms are severe enough to warrant pharmacological treatment. Tricyclic antidepressants, perhaps especially imipramine, have some effect on severe anxiety symptoms, and would be worth trying if there is no evidence of myocardial ischaemia. They should be given in an effective dose for at least four weeks. If they are effective they should be maintained beyond the apparent clinical resolution of the symptoms although the dose may be reduced.

Mrs. A. may be too anxious to tolerate relaxation treatment at first, but teaching her about her symptoms, discussing the kinds of thoughts that precipitate them, and even deliberately evoking them in a demonstration fashion by over-breathing may all help her to regain a sense of control.

Once the initial desperation has subsided, the cause of the anxiety needs to be gone into. Whether the focus is unresolved grief, drug abuse, or conflict about incest that has been evoked by her marriage will depend on the results of further investigation.

Mrs. A. needs to be encouraged to actively engage these problems and to plan for her future as soon as she is able to do so. Her contemporaneous problems should not be neglected. She has few social supports in her new area, and is now unemployed. She may have accumulated some debts. More importantly she has once again been disappointed in her family's ability to care for her. It would be idealistic to suppose that relatives are always well-disposed towards each other, but sometimes family rifts do occur through lack of communication and unrealistic expectations. Efforts should be made, if Mrs. A. is willing, to keep the family involved in her care and, as time goes on, there may emerge an indication for a family meeting in which Mrs. A. would play a much more central role than she believes herself to have at the moment.

Prognosis

It is very likely that Mrs. A' symptoms will remit although, in view of the recent deterioration of her social situation and her continuing disappointment with her family, they may not remit completely as they did previously. Should her anxiety become chronic, she is at risk of depression and tranquillizer dependence.

Even if Mrs. A. recovers from this episode, she will continue to be at risk of anxiety states in the future unless a predisposing factor can be identified and successfully resolved.

ACKNOWLEDGMENT

This chapter could not have been written without Dr George Szmukler, with whom we have discussed the business of formulation and how to teach it over a number of years. It is no longer possible to say which of us was responsible for a particular idea and, although Dr Szmukler did not contribute to the writing of this chapter, our discussions with him have prepared the ground for it.

Further reading

Greenberg M, Szmukler G and Tantam D (1986) *Making Sense of Psychiatric Cases.* Oxford: Oxford University Press

Greenberg M, Szmukler G and Tantam D (1982) Guidelines on formulation. *Bulletin of the Royal College of Psychiatrists 6:* 160–162

Hollyman JA and Hemsi L (1983) What do psychiatrists understand by formulation? *Bulletin of the Royal College of Psychiatrists 7:* 140–142

10

The Case History and Summary

Keith J. B. Rix

THE CASE HISTORY

As soon as possible after admission the trainee should record the full psychiatric history and examination findings using the headings and subheadings listed in Table 10.1. The areas of information covered in the Personal History are shown in Table 10.2. Attention to accuracy, detail and completeness at this stage will make it easier to prepare admission and discharge summaries.

THE ADMISSION SUMMARY

In some hospitals an admission summary is prepared between one and two weeks of the patient's admission. It enables those who become involved in the patient's assessment and care to read about essential features of the patient's history without reading all the written case records. It can be organized according to the headings and subheadings in Table 10.1.

THE DISCHARGE SUMMARY

With appropriate organization, the addition of further information converts the admission summary into a discharge summary (see Table 10.3). This should be prepared within a week of discharge.

The complete typed summary should not usually cover more than two sides of A4 paper and allowance needs to be made for the space taken up by the standard heading on

Table 10.1. Plan for case history and admission summary

Usual headings and subheadings in admission summary	*Optional subheadings in full case history*
REASON FOR AND MODE OF REFERRAL	
HISTORY OF PRESENT ILLNESS	
PREVIOUS MEDICAL HISTORY	
FAMILY HISTORY	
PERSONAL HISTORY	Infancy, childhood, adolescence Education Occupational Psychosexual Menstrual Marital Children Forensic Present life situation
PREMORBID, INTERVAL OR USUAL PERSONALITY	
PHYSICAL EXAMINATION	
MENTAL STATE EXAMINATION	
Appearance	
Behaviour	
Form of talk	
Mood	
Thought content	
Abnormal beliefs	
Abnormal perceptions	
Cognitive functions	Orientation Long-term memory Registration and short-term memory Immediate memory Attention and concentration General information Current affairs Abstract thinking Intelligence
Insight	
Reaction to patient	
INITIAL DIAGNOSIS	
DIFFERENTIAL DIAGNOSIS	

Table 10.2. Areas of information covered in personal history

Infancy, childhood and adolescence
Birth, milestones, temperamental abnormalities, family composition and stability, parental relationship, relationship with parents and siblings, home atmosphere, periods of separation, adolescent behaviour, relations with peers, sports and hobbies.

Education
Age at starting school, standards reached, best subjects, relationships with teachers and pupils, truancy, extracurricular interests, exams passed, age at leaving, details of higher education.

Occupational
Training and apprenticeships, chronological account of jobs with details of nature of work, promotions/demotions and reasons for change, attitude to work, employers and workmates, military record and medical category on discharge.

Psychosexual
Sex information – how obtained, masturbation – attitude towards, fantasies, homosexual and heterosexual experiences, sexual relationships, satisfaction, frigidity/impotence, contraceptive measures, venereal disease.

Menstrual
Age at menarche, preparation for it, attitude towards it, menstrual cycle, regularity, associated psychological and somatic symptoms, pregnancies including miscarriages and stillbirths, age at menopause, attitude towards it.

Marital
Length of engagement(s), circumstances of marriage(s), quality of marital relationship(s), details of divorce(s), extramarital relationship(s), current sexual relationship, age, occupation and personality of partner.

Children
Names, ages, health, personality, attitude towards them.

Forensic
Record charges and convictions, periods in detention centre, youth custody, borstal, prison etc. Outstanding charges.

Present life situation
Area of residence, type and adequacy of housing, living companions, debts, arrears, level of amenities, employment situation, use of leisure time, religious habits, drinking and smoking habits, illicit drug use, social relations, aspirations, plans, ambitions.

Table 10.3. Additional items for converting admission summary to discharge summary

INVESTIGATIONS
TREATMENT AND PROGRESS
FINAL DIAGNOSIS
FINAL FORMULATION
INFORMATION GIVEN TO PATIENT/RELATIVES
FURTHER TREATMENT
PROGNOSIS

most hospital summary sheets. It usually comprises name, address, admission and discharge dates, consultant, etc. For ease of storage by general practitioners, the summary should be typed on the two sides of a single sheet of paper.

For re-admissions, some sections can be reduced to "See summary dated . . . ." or "See summary dated . . . ., in addition: . . . .". However, this formula should be used only for the 'Family History, 'Personal History' and 'Personality' sections and the previous summary cited should be easily located.

In most hospitals the psychiatric discharge summary serves two purposes: it summarizes for the general practitioner details of a patient's admission to in-patient or day-patient status and it constitutes a typed record of the admission for hospital staff who will be subsequently involved in the patient's care. Some consultants prefer to send general practitioners a less formal discharge letter, but the danger in doing so is that, without an established format, vital information may be missed out. Research at University College Hospital, London, has shown that even 'drugs on discharge' and 'follow up' are inadequately described in 10 and 40 per cent of communications respectively. The information least likely to be included is what the patient and relatives have been told.

THE PRELIMINARY DISCHARGE LETTER

The standard 'preliminary discharge letter' used by many hospitals which covers little more than 'diagnosis' and 'drugs on discharge' is often not adequate if the general practitioner is likely to see the patient before he receives a full summary. UCH is experimenting with brief preliminary discharge letters which are sent out within 48 hours of discharge and cover the information regarded as of key importance by general practitioners (physical examination, differential diagnosis, investigations, treatment and progress, further management, prognosis and information given to patient/relatives).

The following notes concern the various sections of the case history and summary. A specimen summary follows. References to general practitioners' views of the usefulness of items and how frequently they are actually included in summaries come from the UCH study.

Reason for and mode of referral

A brief statement of why and how the patient came to hospital, incorporating the principal presenting complaint, e.g. 'depressed and regarded as suicide risk by general practitioner who referred to duty psychiatrist'.

History of present illness

Record the presenting complaints in chronological order beginning with the first experienced or observed change from usual. Where appropriate include verbatim description in the full case history. Timing and duration should relate to the point of admission rather than use actual dates, e.g. 'Eight weeks ago . . . .'. Description of each complaint should include mode of onset and any precipitants, development/course and any factors such as life events or difficulties affecting this, and severity as judged by subjective distress and impairment of normal functions, such as relationships, social life, sex, work or domestic activities, sleep, eating, excretory functions, communication and decision-making. Also include treatment prescribed/received, compliance with treatment, response to treatment, attitude to treatment.

Previous medical history

Comprises general medical as well as psychiatric history. Section begins with episodes of illness or injury (mainly childhood ones) which cannot be dated. Next, episodes documented in chronological order beginning each with patient's age, e.g. 'Age 36 . . .'. Where appropriate, mainly for episodes of psychiatric disorder, details of key symptoms/diagnosis, treatment, duration of episode/treatment, response to treatment, life circumstances (if appropriate) and hospital. Include episodes treated by general practitioner, parasuicides and episodes not treated at all. If history of alcohol/drug abuse/dependence include here. Conclude with statement of current treatment for non-psychiatric disorders.

Family history

In *case history* record full details. In *summary* important features are likely to be current relationships with parents/siblings, reactions to deaths of key relatives, and details of relatives who have suffered from any psychological illness. Record general medical conditions which appear familial.

Personal history

Salient information often recorded under various subheadings in the *case history* (see Table 10.2), but condensed without subheadings in *summary*. Events should be dated according to the patient's age at the time.

Premorbid, interval or usual personality

Avoid technical terms and concentrate on creating a living picture of the patient illustrating points with anecdotes or detailed statements. Aim at describing the individual, not a type. Use information from others as well as self-description. Where a diagnosis of personality disorder is made, this section needs to include sufficient information about impairments and problems resulting from personality characteristics to justify such a diagnosis. It is also important to mention the patient's strengths and assets. Understanding them may be a crucial guide to the patient's capacity to engage in treatment and prognosis. See also Chapter 6.

Physical examination

Section regarded as very important or essential by most general practitioners, but adequately covered in less than a half of summaries studied. Restrict to positive findings and some significant negative findings.

Mental state examination

Summarize main features of initial mental state according to framework in Chapter 6. *General practitioners* do not want a lot of information on this but *psychiatrists* do.

Initial diagnosis

This should be the working diagnosis guiding the initial assessment and care of the patient. Should conform with ICD-9.

Differential diagnosis

Short list of other diagnoses being seriously considered at the assessment stage. Required by most general practitioners but only occasionally included.

Investigations

List negative or normal findings without giving values etc. Positive/abnormal findings require more details. Results of urinalysis most often omitted. This section includes results of psychological as well as physical investigations, i.e. rating scale findings, psychometric test results.

Treatment and progress

Essential component of the summary. Chronological account of the clinical course with events dated from admission (e.g. 'On fifth day . . .'). Document psychological as well as physical treatments. Changes in physical condition/treatment also included. Mention significant changes in mental state. Should be possible for reader to reach own conclusions concerning relationships between treatment and clinical course. Significant changes in medication should be recorded. End with brief account of mental state on discharge so that changes from admission mental state are evident.

Final diagnosis

List psychiatric and non-psychiatric diagnoses using ICD-9 terminology. Diagnostic coding errors by records staff reduced if trainee attaches appropriate code numbers.

Final formulation

Brief formulation explaining diagnosis and/or aetiology as appropriate.

Information given to patient/relatives

Rarely included but required by most general practitioners.

Further treatment

'Drugs on discharge': indicate who is prescribing, advise general practitioner on dose, dosage regime and duration of administration. For other interventions specify who will be responsible. In some cases advise general practitioner what changes to anticipate and what to do if certain changes occur. If out-patient appointment made, indicate date and name of professional concerned.

Prognosis

Required by most general practitioners, but only occasionally included. Avoid brief generalizations like 'good', 'poor' etc. (see p.116). Avoid textbook accounts of prognosis of particular disorder. Say what might happen on basis of course of illness, predictable changes in personal or social circumstances, compliance with treatment, etc.

A SPECIMEN CASE SUMMARY

BULL, John Walter. Age 40

REASON FOR AND MODE OF REFERRAL: Increasing overactivity and disinhibition. Disturbing family and workplace. Sent urgently to out-patients by general practitioner.

HISTORY OF PRESENT ILLNESS: Known manic-depressive. Well when seen in out-patient clinic two weeks ago but noticeably anxious about forthcoming promotion. Ten days ago wife thought more irritable than usual. About a week ago started waking early, getting up and occupying himself around house doing various odd jobs. More cheerful than usual, began making unrealistic plans for extending house and buying neighbour's garden when took up new post. Neighbour no longer on speaking terms. Two days ago wrote cheques for millions of pounds in favour of various charities. Bank staff have phoned to ask wife what they should do about his other cheques. On day of admission sent home from work. Colleagues reported he had been interfering in work of other departments and making suggestive remarks to female staff and customers. Stopped lithium 10 days ago when wife persuaded him to change to a herbal medicine.

PREVIOUS MEDICAL HISTORY

Age 19 – period of depression as student. Successful treatment with antidepressants by Student Health.
Age 30 – admitted STUH. Depressive illness. Responded to ECT.
Age 33 – admitted STUH. Depressive illness. Responded to ECT.

Age 35 – admitted STUH. Manic episode, responded to chlorpromazine but followed by depressive illness.
Age 36 – two admissions STUH with manic episodes. Lithium commenced.
Age 39 – brief depressive episode lasting three weeks, treated with amitriptyline as out-patient.

FAMILY HISTORY: Father manic-depressive, died 64 (CVA) when patient aged 30, normal grief; paternal uncle committed suicide. Youngest of four brothers.

PERSONAL HISTORY: Close family. Very academic. Father, headmaster, set high standards. Older brothers all very successful, patient always being compared with them. Uneventful time at primary and junior school. Moved during third year at Grammar, did not like new school – "too rigid, not enough opportunity for sport". Passed all eight O-levels but most grades lower than expected, father "furious". Describes himself as "rebel" in 6th form – was leader of group which tried to challenge organization of 6th form courses. Left with A-levels in maths, physics, chemistry. BSc in mechanical engineering.

Worked for five years for oil exploration company. Left when married, joined major civil engineering firm. Gained promotion rapidly. Next became Head of Operations for Middle East. Well liked by colleagues.

Married aged 26. Wife, Veronica, three years older, former schoolteacher. A timid, shy person who dislikes company. Like his mother she believes in power of herbal remedies. Frequent arguments about this, particularly in relation to treatment of son's asthma. Son Edward (12) asthma since four, doing well at school. Daughter Julia (10) recently broke leg horse-riding.

Lives in modern detached house. Big mortgage so wife works part-time. She resents this as none of her sisters have to do so. Plays squash (as does wife). Drinks up to six units of alcohol at weekends, rarely drinks in week. Non-smoker since University. Active in parent-teacher association. Strives to be as successful as brothers.

USUAL PERSONALITY: Always active but prone to 'fits and starts'. Sometimes has spells when he would not do what he had promised, but would quickly catch up. His 'slow periods' associated with pessimistic outlook and critical self-examination, but no work impairment. During 'fast periods' very cheerful and outgoing. Popular.

PHYSICAL EXAMINATION: Slightly obese.

MENTAL STATE EXAMINATION: Appearance and behaviour: two

days' growth of beard, hair dyed red and green, would not sit still, wanted to know doctor's first name, expansive gestures. *Form of talk:* increased rate of speech, no pauses, difficult to stop, occasionally broke into song; said "Kipling's cakes are the best, did you read Kipling, doctor?". *Mood:* jovial manner but irritable and near to tears talking about son; described himself as 'full of beans'. *Thought content:* mainly grandiose, e.g. buying neighbour's garden, having charity named after him, returning to 'natural healing'. *Abnormal beliefs:* shareholders are going to make him managing director, totally convinced of this. *Abnormal perceptions:* none. *Cognitive functions:* fully orientated, difficult but not impossible to get attention as kept going off point, no other cognitive deficits. *Intelligence:* above average. *Insight:* believes lithium has suppressed his emotions and present state is 'the natural me'. *Reaction to patient:* some of joviality infectious but soon behaviour became irritating.

INITIAL DIAGNOSIS: Manic depressive psychosis, circular type but currently manic.

DIFFERENTIAL DIAGNOSIS: None.

INVESTIGATIONS: Serum urea, creatinine, electrolytes, TFTs normal.

TREATMENT AND PROGRESS: Treated intially with lithium and chlorpromazine. Behaviour became normal on third day. Remained irritable and lacking in judgement until tenth day. Then became miserable, slow, hopeless and withdrawn. Chlorpromazine stopped. Gradually improved without specific antidepressant treatment and had entirely normal mental state for about five days prior to discharge. During those days used ward groups to talk about anxieties concerning new job. Decided that if it did not work would ask to go back to old job.

FINAL DIAGNOSIS: Manic depressive psychosis, circular type but currently manic (ICD: 296.1).

Brief rebound depressive episode (ICD: 296.8).

FINAL FORMULATION: Typical manic episode in known manic-depressive with cyclothymic personality. Apparently precipitated by stopping lithium but alternative explanation is that news of promotion had precipitated slight hypomania which led him to stop lithium.

INFORMATION GIVEN: Patient and wife know diagnosis and have discussed possibility of children being affected. Lithium treatment has been reformulated in terms of it being 'naturally occurring salt' not so much 'a drug'.

FURTHER TREATMENT:

1. Continue lithium carbonate 1200mg at night, oral – general practitioner to prescribe.
2. For review of progress and treatment, out-patient clinic, appointment sent for 18-11-86 with Dr A Morison.
3. Weekly attendance at ward out-patient group for psychotherapy.
4. Low threshold for admission if hypomanic, family advised to contact Dr Morison's team/duty psychiatrist directly.

PROGNOSIS: Further episodes likely but if continues on lithium may not always need hospitalization. Still wonders if wife right about herbal medicines and so possible may stop lithium again. Has never been suicidal but this cannot be excluded if course of illness worsens.

Further reading

Orrell MW and Greenberg M (1986) What makes psychiatric summaries useful to general practitioners? *Bulletin of the Royal College of Psychiatrists 10:* 107–109

Tyrer P, Alexander MS, Cicchetti D, Cohen MS and Remington M (1979) Reliability of a schedule for rating personality disorders. *British Journal of Psychiatry 135:* 168–174

Section 2
Aspects of Treatment

11

Psychotherapeutic and Behavioural Principles

Frank Margison

DEFINITIONS OF PSYCHOTHERAPY

It is common to see in texts of psychiatry the psychotherapeutic principles separated from the rest of the subject as the 'icing on the cake' requiring attention only as a decoration which brings the history of psychiatric thought to our attention. This chapter takes the opposite view: psychotherapeutic and behavioural principles form one of the pillars on which psychiatry stands – both theoretically and practically. Clearly for these principles to hold such a central position a broad definition of psychotherapy must be taken – not one based just on a set of specific treatment techniques.

Hans Strupp, a major contributor to research in psychotherapy, defines psychotherapy as "an interpersonal process designed to bring about modifications of feelings, cognitions, attitudes and behaviour which have proven troublesome to the person seeking help from a trained professional.". This broad definition highlights the four key elements of psychotherapy as a treatment:

- The therapist-patient relationship is of central importance.
- Therapy aims to modify a wide range of experience and behaviour.
- The recipient has suffered from his difficulties.
- The relationship, whilst often being personal, is also professional.

A similar set of elements can be seen in another definition from a British psychotherapist, Anthony Storr, who sees psychotherapy as "the art of alleviating personal difficulties through the agency of words and a personal, professional relationship.".

The trainee is still bewildered by the huge array of therapies available – each therapy with its adherents. Two complementary frameworks are available. The first is derived from the work of Jerome Frank identifying the common therapeutic factors in all psychotherapies, and the second is derived from Robert Cawley, who divided psychotherapies into different conceptual 'levels'.

Common therapeutic factors

Jerome Frank states the following as common elements in all psychotherapies:

- An intense emotionally charged confiding relationship with a helping person.
- A rationale including an explanation of the patient's distress.
- Providing new information to the patient about the origins of the problems and their possible resolution.
- Hope and the expectancy of help.
- Opportunity for the experience of success in therapy and subsequent feelings of mastery.
- Facilitation of emotional arousal.

Levels of psychotherapy

Psychotherapy can refer to both a specific set of skills following a particular theoretical model or an application of general principles in a wide range of medical and other settings.

Level 1 refers to the positive psychotherapeutic aspects of all doctor–patient relationships whilst Level 2 consists in more demanding but non-specific skills needed by the psychiatrist in everyday practice. Cawley also refers to Level 3 psychotherapy (psychodynamic psychotherapy) and Level 4 (behavioural psychotherapy) (see below).

Format, length, depth and technique

When asked in a clinical examination for a formulation the trainee would still be hard-pressed even with the definitions given above to state succinctly the type of psychotherapy which he or she recommends (see p.113). This is partly because the classification of psychotherapy is confused by distinctions made at different levels of abstraction – for example distinguishing group from individual therapies; psychodynamic from behavioural therapies; and long-term from brief psychotherapies.

It is useful to consider the four minimal parameters which need to be specified to describe a particular type of therapy.

Format

Psychotherapy can take place within a group; with a family (however defined); with a couple; or in a variety of specialized settings such as an art group, a psychodrama group, a 'couples' group; or in a broader setting such as a ward (where the presence of the 'community meeting' may be the focal point of therapy).

Length

Psychotherapy can vary in length from one or a very small number of sessions (usually referred to as crisis intervention); through brief therapy (approximately 8 to 20 sessions); medium-term (20 to 50 sessions); through to long-term therapy (more than 50 sessions). These numbers are arbitrarily chosen and the lengths are not clearly differentiated. Typically short-term therapies will have a fairly specific focus, whereas long-term therapy is usually reserved for situations where the aim is more global personality change.

Depth

At one extreme, therapies of any length and in any format can aim to be *supportive* (that is to maintain functioning at the best level possible through a chronic illness or to minimize the disruption of an acute illness or life event). By definition, supportive therapy does not aim to produce substantial personality change. The therapist aims to identify the best level of previous functioning and the habitual defences and mental mechanisms associated with it. The therapist then tries to help the patient to use the best available (or least damaging) strategies to cope as well as possible.

The term *depth* is used to emphasize the other extreme along this dimension where the therapist aims to bring about increased awareness or 'insight' (typically using psychodynamic principles). The therapist is typically *less directive* here and terms such as exploratory or insight-oriented are often used. However, most therapeutic activity lies somewhere between these extremes. To make exploration possible the person needs to feel supported, and in supportive therapy some understanding and insight into recurrent difficulties usually occurs.

Techniques

The last of the four parameters refers to the specific methods applied whatever the format, length or depth of the therapy. The two most important forms of therapy and their associated techniques are discussed briefly later: exploratory psychotherapy (such as psychodynamic psychotherapy) and prescriptive (such as behavioural and cognitive therapies). There are also many other newer sets of techniques associated with more recent models of therapy, for example art therapy and psychodrama which use creativity and action.

A GENERAL FRAMEWORK FOR PSYCHOTHERAPY

This section addresses the trainee's nightmare when told to "do psychotherapy with Mrs X" without any idea what this means in practice.

The structure of an interview

> "Anyone who hopes to learn the noble game of chess from books will soon discover that only the opening and end-game admit of unexhaustive, systematic presentation, and the infinite variety of moves which develop after the opening defy any such description."
> (Sigmund Freud, 1913 from "On Beginning the Treatment").

It is useful to think of each interview as having a beginning, middle, and end (as for that matter has a whole course of psychotherapy). The initial interview is a special case, but the principles can be applied in any interview. In the opening minutes the therapist is making clear, and setting conditions for, a particular form of conversation. The therapist may be assessing whether subsequent interviews are indicated, achieving or reviewing a particular goal, or initiating a form of exploration where the patient is encouraged to talk freely about embarrassing painful topics.

Beginning the interview

Whatever the style of therapy, certain basics are easily forgotten. In the enthusiasm to get to the 'real business' of therapy it is easy to miss out the beginning and leave the patient unhelpfully confused. Simple points in a first interview like checking the patient knows who you are; how long you have to talk; and the purpose of the interview can easily be overlooked. The way the patient responds to this introduction is itself informative – quiet acquiescence, a concern about details, or obvious apprehension – each says something about the patient's immediate concerns and ways of dealing with anxiety.

Ending the interview

In a first interview it is usual to make a tentative summary of the problem and then to outline a possible plan. Negotiating this is called forming a *therapeutic contract* which ideally involves a statement about all of the following:

- What the main problems are.
- What the focus for therapy will be.
- How these aims will be achieved in the therapy (and any work required outside therapy as is the case in behavioural therapy).
- How many times you will meet.
- For how long.
- When (and how) you will review progress.

Other additional information, for example about confidentiality of records or the use of audio tapes, can be brought in or repeated here.

Although this account is stylized it can be seen that the beginning and end of a session have many similarities across models of therapy. However, psychodynamic therapists may have less formality about the goals specified.

The importance of structure

The attention to detail at the beginning and end of sessions reflects the importance which is given to structure and boundaries, particularly in the psychodynamic therapies. Within unavoidable constraints such as being on-call and being responsible for medical emergencies it is important to arrange a regular setting and a regular time. Even when circumstances force a change in structure the therapist needs to acknowledge that this has happened so that future events such as the patient being late for sessions repeatedly can be understood as a meaningful communication.

Therapist style

Research into the process of psychotherapy has shown systematic differences in style between therapists of different orientations and also that a given therapist can modify his or her style systematically when carrying out different types of psychotherapy. There are also important stylistic differences relating to the personality and idiosyncrasies of the therapist. One of the many difficulties for the trainee is knowing which of these differences may be usefully encouraged as part of a developing personal style and which are avoidable errors of technique which push the interview away from the desired goals.

The next section describes two contrasting styles: *exploratory* and *prescriptive.*

Exploratory therapy

In exploratory forms of psychotherapy the therapist is directive about how the patient can face his anxiety and explore in the current relationship with the therapist painful themes which have been kept out of awareness. The therapist is relatively non-directive about content. It follows that the therapist will ask relatively few questions, but will reflect back to encourage more exploration. There will be relatively little advice and instruction, except to suggest that the patient might "stay with" or explore an area further. The content will focus on relationships from the past and from the present, both outside and within the therapy. The therapist's interventions will often be phrased tentatively and be 'offered' rather than stated dogmatically. The therapist will often link together themes – ways of coping; similarities between relationships; and recurrent symbols. To facilitate this the therapist will actively encourage the patient to explore and develop the capacity to associate freely and to use imagination. This might involve talking about dreams and fantasies or stating thoughts which are usually censored out of conversations. In exploring the meaning of painful symptoms, figurative language like metaphor is encouraged. Often, particular metaphors or 'key phrases' are used to mark a theme for exploration – for example, one patient might frequently refer to themes of 'emptiness' using a word like "hollow".

The whole basis of therapy is thus to seek for personally-relevant understanding whilst symptom relief is seen as a secondary change.

One particular form of exploratory therapy is based directly on psychodynamic and psychoanalytic theory where there is a particular emphasis on *free association* and the use of *interpretation* to allow previously forgotten (repressed) material into awareness. Particular emphasis is placed on *transference* and *resistance* in these forms of therapy. Key theoretical concepts in these forms of therapy are *the unconscious, mental mechanisms, and conflict* (see Glossary and Further Reading).

Prescriptive therapies

In contrast, prescriptive therapies such as cognitive therapy and behavioural therapy focus directly on symptoms and strategies are designed to overcome these. The first stage is to make a detailed analysis of the situations in which symptoms occur more or less frequently *(behavioural analysis)*. This requires detailed questioning of the precise nature of symptoms and requires the strategy of 'funnelling' during interviews, i.e. starting with open-ended questions and following each response with increasingly precise closed questions.

When details have been gathered it is usual to set priorities and then to discuss possible ways of finding solutions. The style of interview is friendly, open and supportive with the therapist acting as a resource rather like a teacher or supervisor. The whole stance in therapy is more distanced from the patient's immediate experience than in exploratory forms of therapy and there is very little reference to the therapist-patient relationship.

The interview will focus on problems that can be expressed clearly. Ideally this will be in a way which allows change to be measured explicitly, often using rating scales and diaries. The therapist will encourage the patient to try out whichever techniques are relevant to the problem. A whole range of techniques are available, all to a greater or lesser extent based on learning theory.

The interview will probably be more structured in the sense that either an implicit or explicit agenda will be followed; for example, starting with a progress report followed by a systematic review and practice of one problem followed by sequential shifts onto subsequent topics.

Traditional behaviour therapy mainly used techniques derived from classical conditioning (for example, systematic desensitization and flooding in phobias, and exposure and response prevention for obsessional symptoms) or operant conditioning (for example, fading and prompting, shaping, time-out, and differential reinforcement of non-problematic behaviours).

More recently there has been growth in three other sets of techniques:

Self-management and skills learning The first relies on the assumption that *self-control can be taught as a set of skills*. The patient *monitors* himself in a systematic way and then sets *specific goals* linked with *self-reinforcement*. *Relaxation* and *anxiety management* can similarly be taught as a systematic set of skills.

Methods based on social learning The commonest example of this, *modelling*, goes outside the general framework of therapist-patient interaction described earlier because here the therapist acts as an appropriate role model in a wide variety of problem areas (for example, in maternal rejection or in overcoming obsessional responses).

Methods based on higher order of learning These all rely on the assumption that unwanted thoughts and feelings can be treated as behaviours. The focus is on problem-solving, for example helping people to manage time more effectively. In cognitive therapies depression and anxiety are seen as the consequences of 'unwanted thoughts' which are then systematically questioned within the therapy. The session will typically end with the setting of homework tasks as well as a summary.

This brief sketch of techniques emphasizes the differences between the two contrasting styles of therapy. In the first, the conversation between therapist and patient *is the vehicle for change itself* whereas in the prescriptive form of therapy the conversation is more accurately seen as the setting through which techniques can be applied more effectively.

As stated above, there is much in common between therapies, but the descriptions show systematic differences in the way the therapist approaches his or her task.

Listening to the interview

The trainee can explore his style in more detail by listening systematically to recordings of his or her own interviews. The therapist is then confronted with four different sorts of information which help in making sense of that interview in the context of his or her own developing skills.

First, the trainee can identify the sort of *interventions* being made (for example, the use of a closed or open-ended question, reflection, reassurance, giving advice or a statement encouraging exploration). This allows the therapist to consider the effect of each type of intervention and whether an alternative might have been better in achieving a particular aim, and pushes the therapist to consider his or her intention behind a particular intervention (for example, to set limits, to gather information, to give information, to improve rapport, to focus or to challenge). Details of the *interventions* are given in Table 11.1.

The second level which can be picked up when replaying an interview is at a higher level of abstraction – the detection of *themes* in the interview reflecting particular areas of *conflict*. Listening to the tape with a chance to pause and reflect allows you to identify core-conflicts, and the way the narrative to the interview changes at times when conflict is

Table 11.1. Interventions

TYPES OF INTERVENTION
(*'What* was I doing?')
(from Shapiro DA, Barkham M and Irving DL (1984) The reliability of a modified helper behavior rating system. *British Journal of Medical Psychology 57:* 45–48, copyright British Psychological Society)

Questioning
- Closed (eliciting specific information)
- Open (eliciting less restricted information)

Advising
- About behaviour outside sessions
- About the process of the therapy
- About specific tasks (e.g. homework tasks)
- How to reframe a problem

Reflecting
- Re-presenting the patient's message

Exploring
- Expressing guesses about the patient's previously unverbalized thoughts and feelings
- Using metaphor and symbols

Interpreting
- Offering the patient a new view of himself
- Making links between past and present (inside and outside therapy)
- Giving tentative explanations about the origins of difficulties

Reassuring
- Agreeing
- Acknowledging
- Supporting and praising
- Sympathizing and stating understanding

Disagreeing
- Pointing out discrepancies
- Giving warnings of unforeseen consequences

Negotiating
- Agreeing a focus for future sessions
- Working towards a shared understanding

Self Disclosure
- Generally about therapist's life (rare)
- About feeling in session

Other
- Talking socially
- Fixing appointments

TYPES OF INTERVENTION
(*"Why* did I do it?")
(from Hill CE and O'Grady KE (1985) List of therapist intentions in a case study and with therapists of varying theoretical orientations. *Journal of Counselling Psychology 32:* 3–32, copyright American Psychological Association)

Structural
- To set limits or make arrangements
- To gather information
- To give information
- To agree a contract/homework etc.

Interview progress
- To support or build rapport
- To focus
- To clarify
- To give hope
- To relieve tension or unhappy feelings

Therapy progress
- To reinforce change attempts
- To overcome obstacles to therapy
- To challenge

Linked with prescriptive therapy
- To identify maladaptive thoughts or behaviour
- To encourage self-control
- To build more appropriate cognitions or behaviours

Linked with exploring therapy
- To identify, intensify and/or encourage acceptance of feelings
- To stimulate understanding or insight

To relieve the therapist's feelings

---

emerging. For example, the conversation may have more pauses, more hesitation, and more markers of heightened feelings in the patient's tone of voice (sounding choked, frightened, etc.).

Malan describes a succinct way of conceptualizing conflict as two simultaneous *triangles of conflict*. One of these refers to the three principles of defence, anxiety, and hidden impulses present in any conflict whilst the other triangle refers to the three main settings where these conflictual themes are repeated – in past relationships, in relationships outside therapy, and in the relationship with the therapist. Even more simply, a conflict can be seen as a wish for something and the simultaneous fears which emerge preventing the wish from becoming reality.

The third level which emerges during the replaying of an interview is the *therapist's own emotional response*. Kagan describes two basic fears which affect people – the threat of engulfment and non-existence, and the threat of alienation and loneliness. Specifically in psychotherapy interviews these emerge as fears of being attacked or attacking, or as fears of being seduced or seducing. Most beginning therapists are quite shrewd and perceptive in picking up these feelings, particularly on replaying an interview. However, beginning therapists are often extremely cautious about relaying these conjectures. This sometimes leads to a 'feigned naivety'. The therapist plays his cards close to his chest and is wary of exposing any uncertainty for fear of the supervisor's contempt, laughter, attacks or distanced non-understanding. Alternatively, the trainee will often think that his or her observation is "too simple" to be worthy of comment in the rarified atmosphere of a supervision setting.

A very useful way of preparing for supervision or studying any psychotherapy session in more detail is to replay an audio tape jotting down the tape counter number and some of the key phrases used by the therapist or patient whilst at the same time noting what is happening at each of the four levels outlined above, i.e. what the therapist's intervention was; what the intention was behind saying it; the nature of the underlying conflict being explored; and the therapist's feeling at that point in the session. This initial analysis of a session allows the therapist to feel more confident in any subsequent supervision and also to be better prepared to listen accurately in the next session.

COMMON THERAPEUTIC SITUATIONS

What can go wrong?

Psychotherapy researchers use the jargon "negative changes induced by psychotherapy" to draw attention to the fact that things can go wrong – a worsening of symptoms; psychosis; aggression; worsening social adjustment; and suicide attempts. Sometimes patients at high risk are offered psychotherapy because the alternative of no treatment is even worse. The factors which predict negative effects include patients who are markedly self-critical and who lack psychological mindedness. Therapist factors include remaining cool and aloof, being insensitive to the patient's state, not providing clear goals and failing to take any responsibility for the course of sessions. In group psychotherapy, casualties occur most often with highly charismatic leaders who set high expectations for their group without providing the means for achieving these and who then make critical remarks to specific group members.

'Setting limits' and coping with emergencies

Many situations occur in psychotherapy where the normal boundaries of the session are under threat. These include inappropriate demands for medication; extreme demands for reassurance or help beyond that initially agreed; telephoning and contacting the therapist between sessions; setting special conditions; criticizing the therapist or his predecessors; quoting what other doctors have said; threats about self-destructive behaviour; and occasionally even blackmail or threats of physical violence.

Murphy and Guze in a paper on 'setting limits' discuss the importance of limit setting in various of these situations. They point out two key principles: (1) maintaining consistency of limits and boundaries, and (2) even when limits have broken down, the therapist not feeling powerless. They point out that the therapist, even when he has made a mistake, can re-establish limits and even use the event to confirm their general importance.

Sometimes the therapist has to rely on his or her personal resources when feeling completely unsure how to cope with a crisis. An example might be a patient suddenly faced with a tragedy like the death of a child. There are no absolute rules to deal with these situations, but most experienced therapists are clear that a 'normal' human response is appropriate, even if it seems to break the rules.

Feeling swamped

At times when dealing with feelings of grief, loneliness, and despair, similar feelings arise in the therapist. The therapist may feel unable to respond as a result of his own feelings or in the belief that no response could be adequate in the face of such overwhelming distress. Again there are no rigid rules or guidelines, but it is worth remembering that even apparently trivial statements like "that sounds awful – it upsets you a lot" or even silence can communicate that you are listening and that the patient is not alone.

It is clear from these comments that psychotherapy can be disturbing. Several authors have noted that the therapeutic process can bring about feelings of personal vulnerability in the therapist, particularly when he or she is working with severely disturbed patients.

Supervision allows the therapist to make sense of these disturbing events, both at a personal level and from a theoretical viewpoint. Even when a trainee is unfortunate enough to have no supervision available, much can be done by talking through sessions with close colleagues or by listening systematically to tapes of sessions.

Further reading

Brown D and Pedder J (1979) *An Introduction to Psychotherapy. An Outline of Psychodynamic Principles and Practice.* London: Tavistock

Frank J (1971) Therapeutic factors in psychotherapy. *American Journal of Psychotherapy 25:* 350–361

Hobson R (1985) *Forms of Feeling. The Heart of Psychotherapy.* London: Tavistock

Kagan N (1980) Influencing human interaction: eighteen years with IPR. In Hess AK, ed. *Psychotherapy Supervision: Theory, Research and Practice,* pp.262–283. New York: Wiley

Malan D (1979) *Individual Psychotherapy and the Science of Psychodynamics.* London: Butterworth

Murphy GE and Guze SB (1960) Setting limits–management of the manipulative patient. *American Journal of Psychotherapy 14:* 30–47

Robertson I (1984) Behavioural psychotherapy. In McGuffin P, Shanks MF and Hodgson RJ, eds. *The Scientific Principles of Psychopathology,* pp.383–408. London: Grune and Stratton

Storr A (1979). *The Art of Psychotherapy.* London: Secker and Warburg

— 12 —

Prescribing and Pharmacotherapy—1

R. H. S. Mindham

Drugs have come to occupy a most important place in the treatment of psychiatric disorders. A generation after the introduction of many of the main types of drugs it is easy to forget or underestimate the effect drug treatments have had in the management of some of the most severe and disabling of psychiatric illnesses. Drugs have come to be taken for granted and even used casually. Whilst drug treatments are not applicable in the whole range of psychiatric disorders, and in some cases are only a part of treatment, the correct employment of drug treatments is of major importance in the work of the large majority of psychiatrists and also important in the work of other medical practitioners who deal with psychiatric disorders. The account which follows is a guide to the use of drugs in psychiatry but is not a full account of psychopharmacology. For details of the drugs available, dosage, and unwanted effects, the reader is referred to the BNF.

CLASSIFICATION OF DRUGS USED IN PSYCHIATRY

In spite of the very large number of drugs available for use in psychiatric disorders, they fall into a relatively small number of major categories which share the same major characteristics. As in other fields no truly satisfactory method of classifying psychotropic drugs has been devised, but nevertheless those classifications available are of great help in understanding and using them. Some of the approaches used in classification will be briefly outlined.

Traditionally in pharmacology, drugs acting on the central

nervous system have been divided into those which enhance or stimulate activity, and those which reduce or depress activity. These two major categories include a large proportion of the drugs which are used in psychiatry. The drugs which have a stimulant effect on the CNS include the antidepressant drugs of the earliest types, such as the amphetamines, to those in current use, such as the monoamine oxidase inhibiting drugs and the tricyclic antidepressants. Drugs which have a predominantly depressive effect on activity in the CNS include the major tranquillizers or antipsychotics and the sedatives. This distinction is an over-simplification in many ways; it is evident that the 'stimulant' effect of amphetamines and of tricyclic antidepressants is different in many respects, as is the 'depressant' effect of antipsychotics and sedatives. Nevertheless, the distinction between the categories has considerable utility. More important, some drugs used in psychiatry fit into neither category; these include the drugs which in a small dosage regularly produce psychotic states, such as mescaline, lysergic acid, and psylocybin and known as the psychotomimetic drugs; and a range of drugs which fit into no group satisfactorily and have to be accommodated in a miscellaneous category; this includes such diverse substances as β-adrenergic blocking drugs and lithium carbonate.

An alternative system for classifying drugs is to label them according to their main therapeutic uses. This system is widely used in books on therapeutics, and can have considerable advantages in certain circumstances because of its immediate clinical relevance. Such a system is heuristically very limited, and is particularly unsatisfactory where a group of drugs has more than one major use.

Chemical names as a basis for classification at least have the virtue of accuracy, but have major disadvantages for clinicians and for pharmacologists. The names of drugs are often cumbersome, difficult to remember, give little or no indication of the likely pharmacological or therapeutic effects, and conversely, drugs with widely differing formulae may have similar pharmacological effects. For these and other reasons chemical names have not been widely used by clinicians, and their contractions to official names are little more helpful.

Alternatively, drugs may be characterized by their pharmacological effects at a cellular level; examples of this are the monoamine oxidase inhibiting drugs or the β-adrenergic blocking drugs. In certain circumstances this approach may have great advantages, especially where the pharmacological effects are thoroughly established and are typical of the group of drugs. With many types of psychotropic drug the situation is less straightforward; there may be diverse pharmacological effects, as is the case of the phenothiazine drugs; there may be uncertainty as to the main pharmacological effects; and occasionally, although the therapeutic effects of a drug may be attributed to a particular pharmacological effect, this relationship may be uncertain or not the only possible mechanism acting in clinical use.

On account of these difficulties a general pharmacological classification of the drugs used in psychiatry is that most widely employed. This has the advantage of grouping drugs together in a way which is clinically useful without being misleading, or prematurely dogmatic about the mechanisms of actions of drugs.

The trainee embarking on a psychiatric career is recommended to view drug treatments in this way; to adopt one of the simple systems of classifying the drugs in use and to think of drugs as members of groups which, while differing in some respects, share many properties. This approach makes the comprehension of drug treatment simpler, makes rational treatment more easily planned, and helps in remembering the likely unwanted effects which patients may experience.

DIAGNOSIS AND EVALUATION

The rational use of drugs, as with other treatments, is dependent upon careful evaluation of the patient's problems.

History-taking, the examination of the mental state, diagnosis and formulation, are dealt with elsewhere, but it should be stressed here that these procedures are essential to the proper use of drugs.

Details of mental state, physical examination, formulation, and the drugs used should be carefully recorded so that the case may be reviewed by others with the full understanding of the reasons for a particular diagnosis having been made, some indication of the reasons for the choice of particular treatments, details of drug dosage and the period of administration, and the outcome of treatment as reflected in changes in the mental state and social functioning. Unless this is done, doctors who may care for a patient in a later episode may not be able to follow the reasons for diagnosis, the rationale in management, or assess the efficacy of treatment.

Psychiatric disorders are often difficult to diagnose or evaluate early in their course, they commonly evolve over a period of years, possibly in successive episodes, and occasionally a change in diagnosis seems necessary to take account of new developments. Patients should be reviewed in detail in successive episodes and the records should be such as to allow this to be done subsequently.

Drug treatments may change the patient's symptomatology and behaviour in ways which will make the diagnosis more difficult or even impossible. Except in the most urgent circumstances patients should be fully assessed and investigated before drug treatment is commenced. This should include assessment of the patient himself, a period of observation where appropriate, the collection of information from informants, including both staff and relatives, and the institution of any investigations which may be necessary (see Chapter 8). Only then should drug treatments be given, unless there are pressing reasons for doing otherwise. It is particularly important that patients suffering from a first mental illness are fully assessed before treatment is begun.

Occasionally a patient will be so disturbed as to require immediate medication to reduce the degree of disturbance, to reduce the risk of harm to the patient and possibly others, and to facilitate nursing and other aspects of care. In these circumstances the details of presentation should be fully recorded, together with a comprehensive account of the mental state, however fragmentary an examination is possible. The evolution of the disorder in subsequent days and weeks may make up for a lack of information at the time of presentation and of emergency treatment.

Very great caution should be exercised in the prescription of antipsychotic drugs for the first time. Unless the period of administration is very short, the institution of antipsychotic therapy is a most significant event in a patient's medical history and the use of antipsychotics will suggest to others that the patient suffers from schizophrenia. Not only is schizophrenia a serious illness with important consequences for work, education, marriage and parenthood, but the prolonged use of antipsychotics carries the risk of the development of tardive dyskinesias, which are often persistent even after antipsychotic drugs have been stopped for many years. Antipsychotics are also particularly likely to change the clinical picture and obscure the correct diagnosis. As antipsychotics are frequently given for long periods it may be years before a condition, not correctly diagnosed in the first episode, is finally elucidated.

Response to medication is very important in assessing the efficacy of treatment, but is of very limited value in establishing diagnosis. An over-hasty use of medication cannot be justified as a 'diagnostic test' in psychiatric disorders.

PLANNING OF THERAPEUTIC REGIMENS

Every patient's treatment should be a carefully planned combination of a range of procedures. The precise plan will depend on the nature of the patient's problem, the patient's social circumstances, the methods of treatment available, and the need to care for the patient during treatment to prevent self-injury and other complications of mental illness. Drug treatment is often a part of a treatment programme especially for patients admitted to hospital. The use of drugs should never be casual, however, and they should always be given with particular effects in mind and the patient subsequently observed carefully to see whether these effects are achieved.

In medical treatment generally methods and drugs vary as to the specificity of their effects. Some treatments have the power to reverse pathological processes or to substitute for a naturally secreted substance which is inadequate; other treatments are non-specific and may suppress symptoms until natural evolution of an illness leads to recovery.

Among the drugs used in psychiatric disorders there are those which may be regarded as having specific effects in the course of an illness, but the great majority simply give symptomatic benefits. The antidepressant drugs may be regarded as having specific effects, although there is uncertainty as to whether they alter the course of a disorder underlying the symptoms or simply suppress the symptoms, albeit fairly specifically, until a natural resolution of an underlying process takes place. Similarly, antipsychotic drugs have a specific effect on dopaminergic neurotransmission which leads to the control of some of the symptoms of schizophrenia, although probably not influencing a more fundamental change. Most other drug treatments are entirely non-specific and these include the sedatives and the hypnotics. The prescriber should have a clear idea why he is using a particular drug and whether a specific or non-specific effect is sought. Some of the drugs used in psychiatry may be used both for their specific and non-specific effects; this is particularly true of the antipsychotics where the drugs display a wide range of actions.

Drugs can only be properly prescribed when the prescriber has a thorough knowledge of the characteristics of the various types of drug available. Most psychotropic drugs need to be given for some time before their main effects in mental illness are seen. The tricyclic antidepressants must be given in appropriate dosage for two to three weeks before the first therapeutic effects are seen, and increasing improvement may be seen to continue even after six or eight weeks. As a consequence, a tricyclic drug cannot be said to have been given a thorough trial in less than four weeks. The main effects of antipsychotics are similarly delayed. Equally important, the effects of withdrawing antipsychotic drugs from a patient whose schizophrenic symptoms are controlled by antipsychotics, may only be seen months afterwards. The dosage of drugs is also important; there is a marked individual variation in the optimum dosage of psychotropic drugs required. An often repeated rule in prescribing psychotropic drugs, but one which is often ignored, is that *they must be given in an adequate dosage for an adequate period of time.*

CHOICE OF DRUGS

The choice between the main classes of drugs will depend upon the diagnosis and formulation. Beyond that the choice of an individual drug in a particular class may depend on a feature of the clinical presentation, such as agitation in depressed subjects, or on the unwanted effects of medication and general acceptability to the patient, but more often on the personal preferences of the prescriber. In general it is better to become familiar with the use of a small range of drugs rather than to use a much wider range very infrequently.

When drugs are ineffective it is common practice to change the treatment. This should only be done when the treatment of first choice has been given a thorough trial according to its characteristics. If it is necessary to change a drug after only a few days, this only suggests that the initial assessment and decision to use it was unsatisfactory. Partial recovery may make assessment during the course of treatment difficult and it is better, once a thorough assessment has been made, to follow through the original choice of drug resolutely.

When it has to be recognized that a drug is ineffective in spite of a thorough trial, a careful note should be made that this has been done, as the experience may serve as a useful guide to future treatment. In choosing a new drug treatment it is then wise to choose one which is different in some respects from the one discarded; for example, a tricyclic drug may be chosen from a different chemical series as in changing from imipramine to amitriptyline, rather than imipramine to desipramine or clomipramine. Alternatively, a totally different drug might be used as in changing from a tricyclic drug to an MAOI. The particular choice will depend on clinical and pharmacological considerations, which are beyond the scope of this chapter.

Most psychotropic drugs are rapidly and completely absorbed from the gut and for this reason oral administration is the method most commonly used. Occasionally, there are advantages in using other routes of administration. In violently disturbed patients, intramuscular injection of an antipsychotic or a benzodiazepine may be the only practical approach. When given by this route drugs are often more quickly and more fully absorbed and the therapeutic effect is quicker in onset. Furthermore drugs given by this route pass into the blood stream largely unchanged and may have a greater effect. Drugs given orally may undergo metabolism in the gut or liver and enter the blood stream as a mixture of the original drug and a range of its metabolites. There are very few indications for intravenous administration of psychotropic drugs; in violent patients this may be impracticable if there are insufficient staff to restrain the patient. Antidepressant drugs are occasionally given by intravenous infusion, but this is not of great advantage therapeutically and is not a widely practised method of administration. Anticonvulsant drugs may occasionally be given by intravenous injection with advantage, especially in the speed of action of the medication. The administration of depot preparations by intramuscular injection is a special case, as this is done to improve compliance rather than to give a rapid effect.

UNWANTED EFFECTS

Unwanted effects are almost always produced when drugs are given in therapeutic dosage. These are largely unavoidable, but as in other branches of medicine, a judgement has to be made as to whether or not the therapeutic effects likely to be produced are greater than the discomfort and risks from unwanted effects. Although therapeutic and unwanted effects may not bear a linear relationship, unwanted effects are a useful guide in judging when a patient is receiving a pharmacologically active dosage of a drug.

Patients should be warned of some of the most common unwanted effects and staff should look out for the more serious effects so that they may be countered by stopping treatment or by other means. Prescribers should be particularly aware of the likelihood of dangerous interactions with other drugs, with food, and of possible effects on the course of physical illnesses from which the patient may suffer. The main interactions are clearly laid out in the BNF.

Some unwanted effects may be diminished by the administration of other drugs, e.g. the use of anticholinergic drugs to control symptoms of drug-induced Parkinsonism. Anticholinergic drugs can change the mental state and interfere with the therapeutic effects of antipsychotics and should be used with caution.

There have been extensive studies of the relationship between plasma levels of drugs, therapeutic effects and unwanted effects. These have been of great interest, but have not become a routine part of management except in the case of some of the anticonvulsant drugs.

COMPLIANCE WITH TREATMENT

Although doctors have prescribed drug treatments for psychiatric disorders for many years, it is only relatively recently that there has been a general awareness that many patients do not take drugs as prescribed. In both acute conditions and chronic conditions patients take drugs much less regularly than the doctor recommends. Adherence to instructions is best in the treatment of acute, unpleasant conditions where the patient has a high expectation of the treatment being helpful either from previous experience or from an understanding of the rationale by which the treatment is used. Even in acute conditions, many patients stop treatment as soon as symptomatic relief is achieved, even though the doctor may have given clear advice to the contrary. In this setting compliance is related to socio-economic factors and to the level of education of patients; those from higher social groups and with more education being more compliant, possibly on account of a better understanding of treatment. In the case of chronic disease compliance with treatment is much less close. With this knowledge it is scarcely surprising that compliance with treatment in some psychiatric disorders is poor. The implications for management of patients and for the interpretation of the results of trials of treatment are self-evident.

Although the problems of compliance are now better understood the problems the matter poses in treatment are far from being overcome. There are problems in treating patients where the very nature of the illness may impair understanding of the need for treatment, or makes compliance unlikely. There are, of course, special considerations where patients are given drug treatments against their wishes (see pp.212–217). There are also difficulties in judging the degree of persuasion which should be used to encourage patients to take drug treatments where the future course of a condition may be uncertain, where the efficacy of the treatment has not been clearly demonstrated, and where serious unwanted effects are possible.

In order to achieve the best possible compliance the doctor must try to establish a good working relationship with the patient in which the patient feels able to trust the doctor's judgement and to enter freely into an agreement to receive drugs and actively follow a treatment. The nature of the patient's problems as seen by the doctor should be fully discussed with the patient, together with an outline of the treatment proposed. An attempt should be made to enable the patient to understand the rationale of treatment and to recognize why it is recommended and why a particular regimen of drugs is necessary. The time scale of treatment should be outlined; this is often a surprise to patients and they also should be warned that they may feel worse in the short term. It should be remembered that even mentally healthy subjects remember only a fraction of what doctors say to them, that retention of information may be selective, and that psychiatric patients may suffer from conditions which greatly impair the capacity to retain instructions and to act upon them.

The treatment recommended should be discussed with relatives and friends, provided that the patient is agreeable. The importance of taking the drugs regularly should be stressed, together with precautions as regards unwanted effects, interactions with food, alcohol and other drugs, the danger of overdose, and the storage and care of drugs, especially in households which include children.

Regular medication is more likely if a simple drug regimen is recommended. For example one daily dosage at night is especially good, as drugs can be kept at home and relatives may supervise their taking unobtrusively. The number of different drugs should be kept to a minimum; this avoids confusion and makes it more certain that the main therapeutic agent is taken. Drug taking can be checked by asking patients in the out-patient clinic what their current pattern of drug taking is; this both checks and reinforces earlier advice. The presence of unwanted effects may indicate that at least some of the prescribed drug is being taken. Depot preparations of drugs may be appropriate to the management of some patients and may be a convenience to the patient as well as to the staff. They are only applicable where good control of symptoms has already been achieved and fine adjustment of dosage is no longer required.

Compliance with treatment may be improved if some warning of unwanted effects is to be given to patients but without overstating the dangers or failing to emphasize the balance between good and bad effects of medication. Drowsiness and possible effects on co-ordination which may pose problems at work, at home or in driving should be mentioned, together with the likely effects of taking alcohol or other drugs with the prescribed medication. It is best to mention the common unwanted effects and to outline the period during which they can be expected to persist. Very unusual unwanted effects are not usually mentioned specifically.

In the average patient it is not wise to argue with the patient over drug taking, he or she usually knows if the drug is being taken as prescribed and the responsibility for this should be placed firmly on them, provided that they are fit to accept such a responsibility. In very ill subjects admission to hospital is likely to be recommended where problems of compliance are rather different, but nevertheless important.

An aspect of compliance which has received much less attention, but is of great importance, is the degree to which doctors prescribe drugs in compliance with their properties, indications, and requirements in administration. Although it is self-evident that drugs may only be expected to be helpful in patients with certain conditions, that only certain dosages are likely to be effective, and that treatment must be continued for an appropriate period, these requirements are often not fulfilled.

RECOMMENDATIONS FOR PRESCRIBING

Prescribing should always be carried out thoughtfully and, except in unusual circumstances, after full evaluation of the patient. The administration of drugs should be part of a therapeutic plan. The drugs themselves should be carefully chosen after consideration of the nature of the illness, the characteristics of the drugs available, and the patient's previous response to drugs from the points of view of both the therapeutic benefits and unwanted effects. Drugs should be given in adequate dosage for a suitable period of time before the drug is judged to be ineffective and a change is made. Where possible drug treatments should be directed towards changing the underlying condition from which the patient suffers, the number of drugs should be kept to a minimum, and the schedule of treatment should be as simple as possible. Incomplete compliance with treatment is a common problem and steps should be taken to increase the likelihood of the medication being taken as prescribed. Unwanted effects and interactions with other substances are many and varied and may require changes in treatment, a reduction in dosage, or additional drugs to control them.

Further reading

British National Formulary. London: The British Medical Association and the Pharmaceutical Society of Great Britain. (Published twice a year)

Tyrer PJ (1983) *Drugs in Psychiatric Practice.* London: Butterworth

Silverstone JT and Turner P (1978) *Drug Treatment in Psychiatry.* London: Routledge and Kegan Paul

— 13 —

Prescribing and Pharmacotherapy—2

R. P. Snaith

The previous chapter has offered sound advice about the general principles of prescribing drugs. The purpose of this chapter is to draw attention to the pharmacotherapy of specific groups of psychiatric disorders.

The art of prescribing should be carefully acquired. Bad prescribing habits nearly always persist as the doctor, with increasing seniority, is subjected less to the benefits of peer review. The junior trainee by reason of his exposed position in the 'front line' is under, or feels himself to be under, pressure to prescribe. Succumbing to these pressures he may soon begin to think less about what he is doing, a casual attitude develops and yet the present and frequently the future well-being of the patient may depend upon careful initial prescribing.

Two short articles are recommended to trainees for further reading. The first is Blackwell's *Treatment Adherence*. Many doctors naively believe that patients will carry out the instructions given, will take the medicines as prescribed and will always do what their doctor tells them to do. However, this belief is very wide of the mark. Blackwell develops the theme of the essential principles of communication between doctors and their patients and if careful thought is not given to these points at an early stage then the doctor will remain an inept prescriber and a poor therapist. The second article is Michel and Kolakowska's *A Survey of Prescribing Psychotropic Drugs in Two Psychiatric Hospitals*. Its authors draw attention to bad prescribing habits that were found to prevail in hospitals of otherwise good repute; some of the prescriptions bordered on the irrational, such as the administration of two or more drugs having the same therapeutic effect at the same time to the same patient. Two particular points are made:

- Most antidepressant and antipsychotic drugs have sedative effects, so the concurrent administration of sedative drugs is rarely justified.
- Most antidepressant and antipsychotic drugs have long plasma half-lives, and once-daily administration should be employed. If the daily dose is given at night the patient is spared daytime sedation, the further prescription of a hypnotic drug is unnecessary and compliance is increased.

THE PHARMACOTHERAPY OF SCHIZOPHRENIA

Effective pharmacotherapy for schizophrenia commenced with the discovery of chlorpromazine, which rapidly led to the production of similar drugs. Some of these drugs produced more, and some less, of certain types of unwanted effects, especially sedation and toxic effects on the central nervous system (acute dystonic crises and Parkinsonism) and neuromuscular function (akathisia and tardive dyskinesia). Chlorpromazine was followed by many other phenothiazines; then came drugs of other basic molecular structures – the thioxanthenes, butyrophenones and diphenylbutyrophenones. None of these has been convincingly shown to have marked superiority over the original chlorpromazine and some, such as haloperidol have markedly increased toxicity. For many the first choice is thioridazine; it lacks the disadvantage of severe photosensitivity induced by chlorpromazine and it is less likely to induce the distressing neurotoxic effects. The only real advance has been the production of depot injections. The establishment of depot clinics and the consequent more regular supervision has led to greater compliance, improved aftercare and a lower relapse rate.

The too early prescription of antipsychotic drugs to a patient who may be suffering from schizophrenia sometimes carries with it the disadvantage of masking the true diagnosis.

The diagnosis of schizophrenia is one of the heaviest responsibilities a psychiatrist has to undertake. It implies a commitment to prolonged, perhaps life-long, treatment; there are liabilities upon status as regards emigration, insurance, employability and there are implications for marriage and procreation. Many people are admitted to psychiatric hospitals with manifestations of abnormal behaviour which resemble schizophrenia; the origins of such behaviour may be cultural, a viral infection, a reaction to some illicit or medically prescribed drug, or in some cases it may even be deliberately feigned. Extreme or unusual stress or experiences may result in 'psychotic' behaviour. Many people with psychotic symptoms will improve spontaneously after admission to hospital and removal from the source of stress. If an antipsychotic drug is prescribed too early, improvement may be attributed to the drug and the conclusion drawn that the 'diagnosis' was schizophrenia with all its implications. The extremely disturbed behaviour of an acutely admitted individual is best managed with intramuscular amylobarbitone sodium until a firm diagnosis can be made. Antipsychotic drugs should *never* be prescribed merely for their sedative effect.

Once a diagnosis of schizophrenia, whether a first episode or a relapse is established, then a carefully considered plan of pharmacotherapeutic management should be presented with consideration of how this is to be integrated with other therapeutic procedures. This should be explained to nursing staff and steps taken to adhere to it. It may take several weeks before the florid disturbance of a schizophrenic episode subsides and a mistake during this period is to assume that the patient is not responding to the selected drug, to keep changing the medication or, worse still, to add one drug to another. If long-term management is with a depot injection, then it is reasonable to prescribe more rapidly effective oral medication, perhaps selecting a drug with a sedative effect, alongside the depot for the first few weeks. However, a patient should not be discharged from hospital on polypharmacy and there should be a definite plan for reducing and stopping the oral medication before the patient leaves hospital; there should also be a period of two or three weeks after withdrawal to be certain that the psychosis has been stabilized on the depot alone. It is important to increase adherence by explaining to the patient the need for long-term medication once he has recovered insight; the more co-operative patients should be given the choice of maintenance on daily oral medication or a three-weekly injection. Maintenance medication should be with the *minimum effective* dose; too often high doses of medication which were necessary in the acute phase of illness are continued in the maintenance period and this only increases the risk of unwanted effects.

There is no justification for the routine prescription of antiparkinsonian medication. These drugs have their own unpleasant and even dangerous side-effects; they may induce hallucinatory states which confuses the clinical presentation, they are associated with dysmnesic problems, and they are sometimes abused and may even be traded by the unscrupulous patient in the pub or on the street corner. However, a very careful watch should be kept for toxic effects of the antipsychotic drug on the central nervous system (see pp.88–89). The most rapidly occurring is the acute dystonic crisis. The Parkinsonian group of symptoms occurs a little later and the matter of detection requires skilled observation. A fixity of facial expression which may be mistaken for a manifestation of concurrent mood disorder is often the earliest sign. When moderate doses of less toxic drugs are used, there is often no necessity for antidotes to the side effects of antipsychotics. Weekly observation for the restless leg movements of akathisia (literally: not sitting) should be kept and noted; there is certainly no effective antidote for this state, just as there is none for the later occurring tardive dyskinesia. The management is prevention, which depends on moderation of dosage and, whenever possible, a choice of less toxic drugs.

An anhedonic depressive state may precede, accompany or follow the recovery from the acute and more florid schizophrenic symptoms. Its recognition is a matter of the greatest importance since it may incorrectly be regarded as 'post-psychotic personality defect', attributed to the 'negative symptoms' of schizophrenia, or attributed to the antipsychotic drug treatment. Failure to recognize it can lead to ineffectiveness of rehabilitation and there is a risk of suicide. Mood disorder is an integral feature of the course of schizophrenia and if it occurs in the post-psychotic phase then it should be adequately treated by the addition of antidepressant medication; usually such antidepressant medication need not be continued for more than three months and the principles of prescription and withdrawal of the drug are the same as in prescribing for depressive episodes of affective disorder (see below). Prolonged prescription of antidepressant drugs in schizophrenia must be avoided since the antidepressant inhibits the effect of the antipsychotic drug.

THE PHARMACOTHERAPY OF AFFECTIVE DISORDERS

Depressive disorders

'Depression' is an overworked concept, loosely used by the profession and the public, to cover a wide variety of states of misery, grief, pessimism, demoralization, frustration, low self-esteem, apathy. In addition psychiatry has a long tradition of recognizing a particularly severe form of mood disorder in which states of 'depression' may alternate with states of mania or occur alone. The term *affective disorder* is used for these states. They are recognized as being constitutionally determined and respond to physical treatments; in other words they are 'biogenic' (a better term than 'endogenous') rather than 'psychogenic', although it is recognized that stress may precipitate a particular episode. In severe states the term 'psychotic' is used, but Kendell, Lewis and others have long recognized that it is only severity which distinguishes psychotic depressive states from milder states sometimes called 'neurotic' depression.

The problems of the prescriber are not with these severe states, but with their milder variants. Even then, a mild manic (or hypomanic) state is not too difficult to recognize, given a distinct departure from the person's usual lifestyle; but the mild depressive (or 'hypomelancholic') state is not defined in any clear way and inevitably becomes confused with the other states of misery referred to earlier. The danger now is that, without clear guidelines for recognizing the mild biogenic depressive state, effective drug treatment will be withheld from many people, whereas many more will be prescribed drugs inappropriately and suffer harm, not only from side effects, but by being dubbed as sick and classified in the company of the mentally ill. Guidelines for distinguishing biogenic from psychogenic depressive mood disorder are not entirely lacking; many psychiatrists rely upon the so-called 'biological' symptoms of sleep disorder, weight loss and diurnal variation, but these are uncertain guides, especially when the patient suffers from a concurrent physical illness. A better guide is the presence of a persistent state of failure to react with pleasure to formerly enjoyed pursuits of 'anhedonia'. It was on the basis of this ability to react with pleasure, that Gillespie distinguished the so-called 'reactive depression', a term which has now taken on a different meaning, i.e. induced by stress. In order to aid physician and others to distinguish this anhedonic (and possibly drug-responsive) form of mood disorder from other states of unhappiness, the brief self-rated Hospital Anxiety and Depression Scale was devised.

If a biogenic depressive disorder, mild or severe, is diagnosed on the basis of careful evaluation of antecedents, associations, course and symptomatology, then the first line of treatment is undoubtedly one of the wide range of antidepressant drugs. Most psychiatrists prefer to commence treatment with one of the tricyclic group and, as with the phenothiazines, there is no sound evidence that any of the large number of these products is more effective or less toxic than imipramine, the first to be discovered. Medical lore and pharmaceutical promotions claim one or other advantage, but these are not usually substantiated. As with the antipsychotic drugs, the tricyclics have long plasma half-lives and, with the possible exception of the elderly, who may suffer from hypotension if a large single dose is given, and patients with a past history of cardiac disease, there is no advantage in spaced prescribing. A single dose at night will increase compliance and obviate the need for the addition of a hypnotic drug. The repeated mistake in the prescription of tricyclics, as with other antidepressant drugs, is the administration of a subtherapeutic dose, assumption that the drug is ineffective, and change to another medication; this error *must* be avoided and drug treatment should not be declared to be ineffective unless it has been administered in full therapeutic dose for *at least* four weeks. If one tricyclic is ineffective, there is probably no point in changing to another. In fact, if a tricyclic antidepressant drug is ineffective it is unlikely that a change to any other type of antidepressant drug will have an effect unless, of course, it coincides with the natural remission of the illness. There is evidence that the addition of lithium is useful in some cases of resistant depression.

The successful use of drugs depends in great part on how they are prescribed, and in no field is this more true than in depressive states. Many patients resist the concept that their suffering is due to neurochemical imbalance, many are suspicious of 'drugs for the mind', and believe that all such drugs produce dependence. Finally there is the delay of therapeutic effect and the initial discomfort of unwanted effects before this is rewarded by improvement. All this requires careful explanation to the patient, for otherwise non-adherence to the treatment is certain to occur. In order that the patient may adapt most easily to the unwanted effects, it is advisable to prescribe in increasing dose, e.g. imipramine 50mg for the first three days, then 100mg for the next three days, then 150mg, and finally the full dose of 200mg a day.

The major reason for changing from a tricyclic is severe discomfort from the side effects and especially extreme dryness of the mouth, visual accommodation difficulties, difficulties with micturition and severe constipation. If these effects are persistent and severe, then a change to a non-tricyclic such as mianserin or viloxazine may be justified; however, all drugs have their own range of side effects and the prescriber must be acquainted with these; for instance, mianserin has been implicated in toxic effects on the marrow and a routine haematological examination is a reasonable precaution during prescription.

There is some controversy concerning the use of MAOIs in the treatment of depressive disorders. Some regard them as only weakly antidepressant. Others regard them as generally effective and particularly effective in certain patients or conditions: classical severe depression with marked psychomotor retardation; severely depressed, non-deluded in-patients; depression accompanied by apprehension and marked anxiety with impaired concentration, depersonalization and a tendency to blame others; depression with 'reversed vegetative changes' (i.e. *onset* insomnia, hypersomnia, increased appetite, weight gain, increased libido); and significantly depressed patients who fail to respond, or react badly, to tricyclics and ECT. However, the following possible hazards of MAOI treatment have to be considered: hypertensive crises (some serious or fatal), even in patients who meticulously follow their diet and are warned about interactions with proprietary medicines; hypomania; weight gain; erectile or orgasmic dysfunction; withdrawal symptoms; and self-poisoning which is difficult to treat.

If there is failure to respond to adequate antidepressant drug treatment, then the grounds for prescription should be thoroughly reviewed. If the conclusion is still that the depressive state is essentially biogenic then the use of ECT should be considered without further delay; at one time this effective treatment was overused and this contributed to an unfortunate swing against it; now it is probably underused.

The duration of continuation of prescription of antidepressant drugs is a matter of individual judgement. Since the drugs help to lift the mood during a phase of the disorder, stopping medication whilst the patient is still in the active phase will inevitably lead to relapse, but stopping the drug after the phase has ended will not lead to relapse, although a further phase may occur at a later date. All this should be explained to the patient, and it is helpful to draw a simple diagram to make the point clear; a doctor should not be ashamed to admit that he cannot know for certain whether a patient could remain well without the drug, and that a trial of withdrawal is a sensible procedure. There are a few patients who are helped by antidepressant drugs taken over a prolonged period of time, but even so, a trial of withdrawal every year or so is in order. It is now recognized that there are withdrawal syndromes (mainly gastrointestinal symptoms and insomnia) when antidepressants have been taken for a long period of time, and they should therefore be withdrawn gradually over a period of several weeks or longer.

Mania

The treatment of manic attacks is with antipsychotic drugs or lithium. In acute states oral antipsychotic medication is unreliable and medication by injection is usually necessary. In such states a powerful drug such as haloperidol is usually justified, but careful observation for early toxic effects is necessary. Medication need not be prolonged, as with schizophrenia and the same principles of explanation and trial of withdrawal apply as in the case of antidepressant therapy.

The uses of lithium

Lithium is used in the prophylaxis of manic-depressive psychosis and recurrent unipolar depressive illness. It is sometimes used in the treatment of manic and depressive episodes.

Often the prescription of the drug implies long-term therapy and the inconvenience and risks of this are certainly not to be considered until the patient has had at least three, closely spaced, attacks of mood disorder and the attacks are causing increasing disruption of the patient's life and relationships. If pregnancy is to be planned then lithium should be withheld and caution is necessary if lithium is to be given to a patient suffering from renal disease, epilepsy, Parkinsonism or diabetes mellitus. Prior to lithium treatment the following investigations should be carried out: urinalysis, full blood count, ESR or plasma viscosity (PV), serum urea, creatinine and electrolytes, and thyroid function tests. In some patients it may be wise to carry out a lithium tolerance test. The trainee must learn early to recognize the toxic effects of lithium: vomiting, diarrhoea, ataxia, dysarthria, weakness, muscle tremor and twitching. In addition, serum urea, creatinine and electrolytes should be measured and thyroid function tests carried out every six months.

THE PHARMACOTHERAPY OF ANXIETY DISORDERS

Most people who suffer from an anxiety-based disorder and who come to a medical doctor for relief of their distress, are either alarmed about the significance of some symptom such as palpitations and request physical examination or else they hope that a simple pharmacological solution may resolve the discomfort. By long tradition the function of the medical profession is the prescription of medicines and many practitioners still consider that consultation must be followed by prescription of some drug or medicine. The result is an endless dispensation of pills and potions, some harmless, but others less so, which serves only to confirm their recipients belief in their 'sickness'. However, there are some signs of change, since doctors are now receiving better psychiatric education. A second major factor is the growing awareness that harmful effects exceed the transitory benefits of many drugs and this causes increasing demand for a non-pharmacological solution for anxiety-based disorders.

Sedative drugs

Many psychotropic drugs have a sedative effect and, as already pointed out, this sometimes is beneficial in the treatment of psychiatric disorder, but at other times it is an unwanted effect. Generations of drugs have been prescribed solely for their sedative effect. The creation of the present generation of benzodiazepine drugs enabled the medical profession to forego the widespread use of barbiturates and, although reports of physical dependence occurred early in the benzodiazepine era, such was the apparent need for sedative drugs that these reports were widely overlooked. The term 'anxiolytic' was created in the beguiling belief that these drugs reduced anxiety without other effects but, if the matter was overlooked by the medical profession, the pharmaceutical industry was well aware of the basically sedative nature of all the drugs and some were deliberately marketed as hypnotics.

There is growing awareness that benzodiazepines can produce states of true physical dependence. It is now quite obvious that large numbers of people continue to take benzodiazepine drugs over periods of months and years, not because they have any beneficial effect, but because withdrawal often leads to considerable distress. The distress is not simply the recurrence of original anxiety symptoms (in many cases these were never significantly reduced by the drug), but a rebound anxiety of a different quality, severe insomnia and a variable accompaniment of characteristic symptoms: numbness and paraesthesiae, retching and vomiting, hypersensitivity to noise and light, a characteristic sensation of the distortion of the sense of the position of the body in space, hallucinatory experiences and in some cases withdrawal fits. There are now many individuals for whom it must be judged that continued prescription of benzodiazepines is the lesser evil; distress caused by withdrawal is a combination of duration of prescription, type of drug, and personality factors. Certainly there are some individuals who can stop prolonged medication with little distress and the well-motivated person may be encouraged to do so, so long as it is borne in mind that sudden withdrawal after prolonged administration can lead to fits which may put the person at risk.

If benzodiazepines are to be prescribed at all, this should only be for very short courses and after clear explanation of the risk of dependence. Moreover, a warning should be given that the drug will potentiate the effect of alcohol, and so cause the person to be unsafe after a drink that has previously been taken with safety.

Antidepressant drugs

These drugs may be very effective in some patients who present with symptoms of anxiety; this was first recognized soon after the introduction of tricyclic antidepressants when it was observed that states characterized by pervasive anxiety, panic attacks, progressive handicap of the agoraphobic type, sometimes depersonalization and other features, improved remarkably after prescription of the drug. Since the drugs had an already established reputation as 'antidepressants', it was considered that such states were a form of 'atypical depression'; the alternative view is that the drugs are effective over a wider range of *mood* disorder than the term 'antidepressant' implies.

ICD-9 recognizes only one category of anxiety state, whereas DSM-III recognizes a broad distinction between 'General Anxiety Disorder' and 'Panic Disorder'. This distinction rests upon the observation of a number of prominent American psychiatrists that there is a form of anxiety disorder which presents acutely as severe peaking of anxiety (panic attack), accompanied by symptoms of autonomic overactivity and a lack of sufficient stress to account for such a catastrophic episode. At first, attacks may be widely spaced or there may be only one episode, but in many cases increasing pervasive anxiety leads to a wide range of avoiding responses and the emergence of the agoraphobic syndrome. Panic disorder may respond to antidepressants if administered cautiously and at the correct time, that is early enough in the course before avoidance responses have become entrenched. There is some evidence that MAOIs (see p.173) are rather more effective than tricyclic antidepressants but, whichever drug is selected, it is necessary to bear in mind that these highly anxious people are extremely sensitive to side-effects of the drug; if the patient is to comply with treatment it is necessary to commence with an extremely low dose, say 25mg imipramine or 15mg phenelzine daily, and to increase the dose very gradually until a satisfactory therapeutic response occurs.

CONCLUDING COMMENTS

There can be little doubt that the recent era of psychopharmacology has brought great advantages, but also considerable disenchantment and recognized adverse effects. The trainee must learn, at an early stage, to respect these powerful drugs and to write every prescription with great care.

Space does not allow a detailed consideration of many special circumstances. People whose brains are damaged by disease, congenital or acquired, require even greater care in prescribing. For instance patients suffering from dementia or low intelligence are unable to protect themselves against the injurious effects of drugs by complaining of side-effects. In all circumstances, and especially in conditions where the adverse effects of drugs may be increased, the trainee must be careful to seek advice from experienced clinicians and, of course, the Drugs Information Department in the hospital pharmacy.

Further reading

Blackwell B (1976) Treatment adherence. *British Journal of Psychiatry 129:* 513–531

Blackwell B (1986) Monoamine oxidase inhibitors. *British Journal of Psychiatry 148:* 216–217

Michel K and Kolakowska T (1981) A survey of prescribing drugs in two psychiatric hospitals. *British Journal of Psychiatry 138:* 217–221

Pare CMB (1985) The present status of monoaminc oxidasc inhibitors. *British Journal of Psychiatry 146:* 576–584

Snaith RP, James FE and Winokur B (1979) The drug treatment of mental illness and epilepsy in the mentally handicapped patient. In James FE and Snaith RP, eds. *Psychiatric Illness and Mental Handicap,* pp.55–64. London: Gaskell Press

Zigmond AS and Snaith RP (1983) The Hospital Anxiety and Depression Scale. *Acta Psychiatrica Scandinavica 67:* 361–370

— 14

Giving Electroconvulsive Therapy

I. Pennell & J. F. W. Deakin

Electrically induced seizures have been a physical treatment in psychiatry for over 40 years. The first treatment was administered in 1938 by Cerletti, an Italian psychiatrist who had been impressed by the tranquillizing effects of artificial seizures in animal experiments. Use of ECT spread rapidly and psychiatrists who remember its introduction have described the dramatic effects on the chronic in-patient population of the time, for which there had been no effective treatment.

With the development of short-acting anaesthetics and muscle relaxants, unmodified ECT was replaced by modern ECT in which convulsions are attenuated or abolished by the anaesthetists' drugs while cerebral seizure activity is retained. Assertions that modified ECT is less effective than unmodified ECT have no empirical foundation.

The mechanism of action of ECT is not known. In animal experiments, repeated seizure induction causes gradual changes in monoamine receptor systems. It has been suggested that some of these delayed receptor changes may be a common mechanism of action of all antidepressant therapies since they are shared by ECT and most antidepressant drugs.

INDICATIONS AND PREDICTIONS OF RESPONSE

The antidepressant efficacy of ECT has been placed beyond doubt by many clinical trials. It is further established that the passage of electricity is the critical therapeutic ingredient rather than placebo or anaesthetic effects. Recent well-controlled studies suggest that ECT also has therapeutic effects in schizophrenia, but its place in the treatment of schizophrenia is a matter of continuing debate.

Several studies have attempted to relate features of the mental state in depression to subsequent response to ECT. Most studies agree that biological and psychotic symptoms predict a favourable outcome. A widely known predictive scale was developed by Carney, Roth and Garside and it is reproduced in Table 14.1. Whether such scales do more than identify patients with a good prognosis and response to any antidepressant treatment is not clear.

Table 14.1. ECT response prediction scale

(from Carney MWP, Roth M and Garside RF (1965) The diagnosis of depressive syndromes and the prediction of ECT response. *British Journal of Psychiatry 111:* 659–674, with the kind permission of the Royal College of Psychiatrists)

Weight loss of more than 3kg	+3
Pyknic build	+3
Early wakening	+3
Somatic delusions	+2
Paranoid delusions	+1
Worse pm	−3
Hypochondriacal	−3
Hysterical	−3
Anxiety	−2
Self-pity	−1

A total score of +1 or more predicts a good response to ECT
A total score of 0 or less predicts a poor response to ECT

ECT as a first rank treatment

There is evidence that depressive illnesses with biological features respond more rapidly to ECT than to drugs. ECT should therefore be used as a first treatment in depressives who are dangerously suicidal or retarded, where a rapid response is desirable. The presence of delusions is often taken as an indication for ECT and some studies indicate that delusional depression is refractory to antidepressant drugs and particularly responsive to ECT. It is widely held that puerperal psychosis and catatonic stupor respond well to ECT.

ECT as a second rank treatment

ECT is often used in patients with depressive illnesses which have not responded to adequate doses of antidepressant drugs. Severely overactive manic patients who have not responded well to neuroleptic drugs and lithium are sometimes successfully treated with ECT. It has been advocated in the treatment of schizophrenia with marked depressive features, but ECT does not influence the deficit symptoms of schizophrenia and these must be carefully distinguished from depression.

CONTRAINDICATIONS

There are no absolute contraindications to ECT and the risks of the treatment have to be weighed against the risks of conservative treatment. Clearly, it is necessary to determine that the patient is fit to receive a general anaesthetic and acute respiratory infections, other respiratory problems and ischaemic heart disease are relative contraindications. The convulsive shock produces changes in heart rate, a pronounced but usually short-lived rise in blood pressure and an increase in cerebral blood flow. Therefore, extreme caution is necessary where there is CNS or cardiovascular disease and conservative management should be considered in the following:

- myocardial infarction in last three months
- pacemaker patients
- cardiac arrhythmias
- cerebral and aortic aneurysms
- recent cerebral haemorrhage
- raised intracranial pressure and CNS tumours

A routine pre-treatment assessment is shown in Table 14.2. The anaesthetist should always be warned of any medical problems and advised of the patient's drug treatment. It is advisable to stop lithium treatment 48 hours before ECT in view of its interaction with muscle relaxants.

Table 14.2. Pre-treatment assessment

Medical History
Including medication, drug sensitivity, response to previous treatment, family history of drug sensitivity.

Physical Examination
With careful attention to neurological aspects, including the fundi, to the cardiovascular and respiratory systems.

Investigations
Urinalysis
Full blood count
Fasting blood sugar
Blood urea and electrolytes
Chest X-ray
ECG

Sickle cell test for negro patients

Other investigations indicated in individual patients

THE SETTING IN WHICH ECT IS GIVEN

The minimum requirements of a suite where ECT is given are set out in the College Memorandum. The patient should wait in a comfortable waiting room with a nurse in attendance to give reassurance. Separate treatment and recovery rooms should be provided. The ECT room should be staffed by the psychiatrist giving the treatment, the anaesthetist, an experienced charge nurse and two junior nurses. Suction and emergency resuscitation equipment should be readily available.

ANAESTHESIA

With any anaesthetic the patient must be starved of fluids and food for eight hours. ECT is usually administered after an overnight fast. Before anaesthetic induction, the patient's dentures are removed. Table 14.3 shows a sequential drug regime for inducing anaesthesia for ECT.

Table 14.3. Anaesthesia for ECT

1. Atropine 1.0–1.5mg IVI	Dries respiratory secretions, protects against vagal bradycardia
2. Methohexitone 0.75–1.0mg/kg body weight (initial dose) by rapid IVI	Fewer cardiac problems than thiopentone. Rapid injection produces rapid induction
3. Suxamethonium 0.5mg/kg body weight (initial dose) IVI over 1–2 seconds	Dose not so high that the convulsion is completely abolished

(Based on Pitts FN Jr Medical physiology of ECT. In Abrams R and Essman WB, eds. *Electroconvulsive Therapy. Biological Foundations and Clinical Applications.* 1982. Lancaster: MTP Ltd, with the kind permission of Spectrum Publications).

After anaesthetic induction, a mouth gag is inserted to prevent damage to teeth, gums and oral mucosa, and the patient is ventilated with 100% oxygen for a few seconds before the stimulus and after the seizure until the return of spontaneous respirations. This minimizes the risk of hypoxic damage to the CNS and myocardium. Insertion of an airway after the seizure reduces the risk of respiratory obstruction.

The patient is placed in the semi-prone recovery position and moved to a recovery area where a nurse is in attendance. After recovery the patient should return to the ward and be encouraged to sleep.

THE ECT STIMULUS

The ECT apparatus should be of the type that delivers a series of brief pulses of electricity over an automatically timed duration. This design has superseded earlier designs in which a variable part of the sinusoidal AC waveform was used. The brief pulse machines use a smaller quantity of electricity to induce a convulsion than the older designs and this may result in less post-ECT confusion and amnesia.

The Ectron Constant Current machines are the most widely used type in the UK which conform to present electrical standards. The following account of the operation of these machines (Series 2 onwards), is intended as a guide only, and users should always have proper training in their use and read the manufacturer's instructions before administering ECT.

1. Check the electrode pads have been adequately soaked in electrolyte solution.
2. Switch the mains switch to the 'On' position.
3. With the mode set at 'Test', press together the electrodes with their pads soaked in electrolyte solution. A satisfactory circuit is indicated by the glowing Test light.
4. Set the mode at 'ECT 1', and the Time at 4 seconds. This strength of stimulus will induce a convulsion in the majority of patients.
5. Place the electrodes on the prepared patient.
6. Press the electrode switch to administer the stimulus and keep the electrodes in position until the audio signal stops. If a convulsion definitely does not occur, the stimulus may be repeated once or twice at a longer time setting or with the mode set at 'ECT 2', but if after three attempts there is still no convulsion, allow the patient to recover in the normal way and request in the case records that the procedure be reviewed.

NB The 'Auto Crescendo' switch on the Constant Current machines allows the current to build up over 0.5 seconds, inducing a gradual tonic phase. Its use is optional. Some

Ectron machines ('Ectonustim') have a 'Cerebral Stimulation' facility which delivers a subconvulsive electrical stimulus. This has no place in electroconvulsive therapy.

PLACING THE ELECTRODES

To ensure good contact between the patient and the electrodes, the relevant areas of skin should be rubbed with electrolyte solution, and if the skin or hair is greasy it should be cleaned beforehand with a swab soaked in alcohol.

The electrode pads are placed in electrolyte solution when they are not being used.

It is desirable to use two individual electrodes allowing firm pressure to be exerted with each hand. One electrode contains a switch to deliver the stimulus. Pairs of electrodes which are held in one hand do not guarantee good electrical contact with the skin.

Various electrode positions have been advocated and Figure 14.1 shows positions recommended by the College. For bilateral ECT the pads are pressed to the temporal fossae at a point approximately 4cm above the mid-point of a line joining the external angle of the eye and the external auditory meatus (Figure 14.1a).

For unilateral ECT, the positions are shown in Figure 14.1b. The patient's head should be turned to one side to allow firm downward pressure to be applied to both electrodes. The lower electrode is placed as for bilateral ECT, over the non-dominant hemisphere (usually the right, see below), and the upper electrode 12cm away above and behind the ear.

OBSERVING THE CONVULSION

A few seconds after the muscle relaxant is given, widespread fasciculation indicates that the muscles are depolarized and

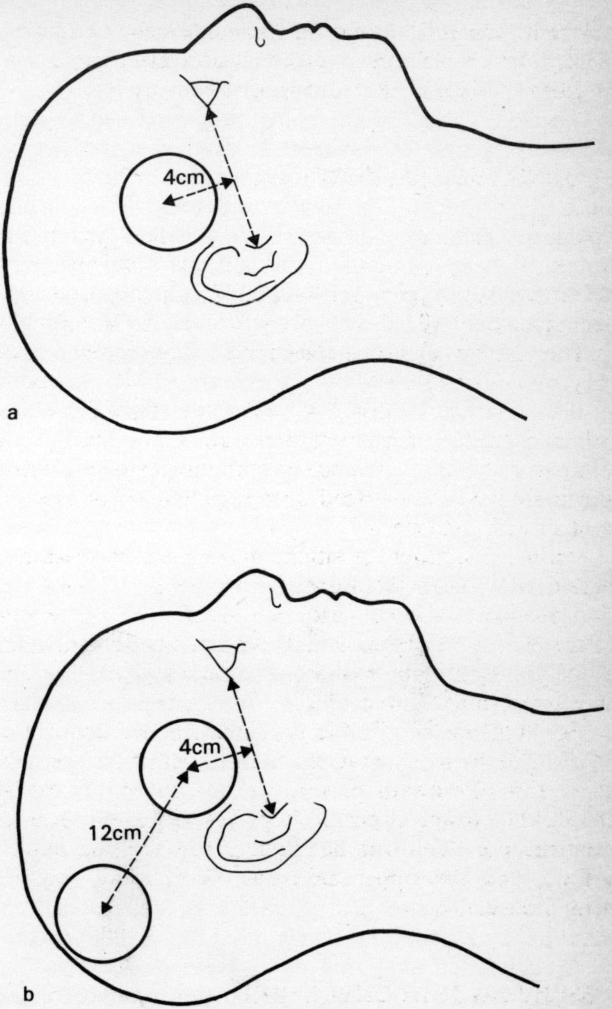

Fig. 14.1. Electrode positions recommended by the Royal College of Psychiatrists for bilateral (a) and unilateral (b) electroconvulsive therapy.

paralysed. Immediately the ECT stimulus is started a powerful tonic jerk occurs due to direct electrical stimulation of the cortex. This is not the therapeutic convulsion.

The clonic phase of the convulsion, modified by muscle relaxant, appears several seconds after the stimulus, and consists of mild rhythmic contractions, which are best observed in the eyelids, fingers and toes. The convulsion should be bilateral, following both unilateral and bilateral stimuli. If there is doubt whether a fit has occurred, perhaps due to excessive muscle relaxation, on subsequent occasions a sphygmomanometer cuff inflated to above systolic blood pressure on the opposite arm to that in which the muscle relaxant is given will allow observation of an unmodified convulsion in that arm.

Benzodiazepine night sedation is best avoided the night before ECT. Residual drugs may attenuate the therapeutic convulsion.

RECORDING THE TREATMENT

A record of each application should be kept in the patient's file. The date, details of anaesthetic drug dosage, ECT machine settings and details of the convulsion should be recorded. Comments on any complications and recommendations for the next application should also be recorded.

NUMBER OF APPLICATIONS

Most patients receive 6–8 applications, some patients respond to 2–3 and others may need 10–12. Applications are usually given at a rate of 2–3 per week. There is no evidence that more frequent application produces a faster response.

ASSESSING CEREBRAL DOMINANCE FOR UNILATERAL ECT

Unilateral ECT is almost as effective as bilateral ECT in the treatment of depression, although some studies suggest that slightly more unilateral treatments need to be given.

Unilateral ECT applied over the non-dominant hemisphere for language certainly produces less verbal memory impairment and post-ECT confusion than bilateral ECT or unilateral ECT over the dominant hemisphere. These findings account for the growing use of unilateral treatment. It is therefore necessary to determine which hemisphere is dominant for language in a patient who is to receive unilateral ECT.

In predominantly right-handed people, over 90 per cent are language dominant in the left hemisphere, but in the case of left-handed people and ambidexters, over 50 per cent are also language dominant on the left, only 40 to 50 per cent being right dominant. Left handedness is therefore a poor guide to cerebral language dominance, and a further assessment of dominance should be carried out in these patients.

Handedness can be reasonably reliably ascertained by asking the patient which is the preferred hand with which to write, throw and use a tool. For strongly right handers, unilateral ECT should be given on the right side. Right handers who suffer confusion or who complain of memory difficulties after one treatment can be further assessed according to the procedure for left and mixed handers.

For these patients, a simple test of word-finding is given after right and left unilateral treatments.

The test consists of four questions which are given as soon as the patient is able to respond correctly to the question: "What is your name?". Table 14.4 shows the questions, with a convenient format for recording the correct answers.

In the majority of cases, patients will give fewer correct answers on one occasion than the other, and this indicates the hemisphere dominant for language. Subsequent ECT should be given on the side for which most correct answers were given.

Table 14.4. Assessment of dominance

Question	Correct answer after ECT to right side (tick)	Correct answer after ECT to left side (tick)
1. What is the thin, grey dust which remains after something is burnt, like a cigarette? Answer: Ash 2. What is the hard outer case which protects animals like tortoises and snails? Answer: Shell 3. What do broadcasters speak into so that they can easily be heard? Answer: Microphone 4. What is the glass or polished surface into which one can look and see a reflection of onself? Answer: Mirror		
Number of correct answers		

(from Pratt RTC and Warrington EK (1972) The assessment of cerebral dominance with unilateral ECT. *British Journal of Psychiatry 121:* 327–328, with the kind permission of the Royal College of Psychiatrists).

SIDE EFFECTS AND COMPLICATIONS

ECT is safe. The mortality rate is similar to dental anaesthesia and in a large series the rate was approximately one death per 20,000 treatments. The rare physical complications are:

- anaesthetic complications
    - cardiac arrest and arrhythmias
    - pulmonary embolism
    - pneumonia
- insufficient muscle relaxation
    - dislocation
    - fracture and fat embolism
- ECT induced blood pressure rise
    - bleeding peptic ulcer
- prolonged seizure requiring intravenous anticonvulsants
- spontaneous fits

The psychological complications are the precipitation of mania in approximately five per cent of cases and cognitive impairment. Post-ECT confusion usually lasts half an hour but may occasionally be longer-lasting. Psychological tests show a short and rapidly decreasing retrograde amnesia and a degree of anterograde amnesia for approximately 24 hours after each treatment. Many patients are unaware of these effects and depression itself is associated with cognitive impairment. In a large series, no cognitive impairment could be demonstrated a month after a course of eight ECTs. However, some patients complain of persistent difficulty recalling remote personal memories months or years after ECT. Research has not so far established whether such complaints are genuinely attributable to ECT or to other factors such as continuing depressive illness.

Headaches occur frequently and may occasionally persist for some hours. They may be caused not by ECT itself, but by the muscle relaxant.

CONSENT TO ECT

The principles of consent in England and Wales are discussed in the Mental Health Act Commission's draft document 'Consent to Treatment' issued for discussion in July 1985.

Except under special circumstances, ECT can be administered only after written consent is given by the patient. The trainee and nursing staff must confirm that written consent has been obtained.

The treatment must be explained in broad terms to the patient. The amount and detail of information given will vary from one patient to another, but should include discussion of the following areas.

The patient should have an idea of the procedure and number of treatments. Reference should be made to the small but definite risk that all anaesthetics carry, especially if the patient is at risk of medical complications. The patient should know about the likelihood of headaches and temporary and longer-term memory problems.

In general, definite assurances of a particular result or absence of risk should be avoided, as the doctor is seldom in a position to make such assurances.

Mention should be made of alternative treatments which are available, with their attendant risk and likely outcomes, as well as the likely outcome if no treatment is received.

The patient should be given the opportunity to air questions or worries about ECT, and these answered honestly and openly. A full explanation should also be given to the patient's nearest relative.

The signed consent form should be prominently displayed in the notes, preferably on the same form used to record the treatments.

ECT may be given to patients detained under Section 3 of the Mental Health Act, but there are special requirements about consent and a second opinion may be a statutory requirement.

Further reading

Kendell RE (1981) The present status of electroconvulsive therapy. *British Journal of Psychiatry 139:* 265–283

Palmer RL, ed. (1981) *Electroconvulsive Therapy: An Appraisal.* Oxford: Oxford University Press

Pippard J and Ellam L (1981) *Electroconvulsive Treatment in Great Britain, 1980.* London: Royal College of Psychiatrists

Section 3
Special Topics

15

Patients from Other Cultures

Philip H. Rack

Britain is multicultural and multiracial. In every industrial city the population includes some people who were born in other countries and they are at least as likely as others to become psychiatric patients. Any psychiatrist may be consulted from time to time by a patient whose attitudes and lifestyle are different and unfamiliar. Unless cultural factors are understood, accurate diagnosis is impossible and treatment is unsatisfactory.

When you meet such a patient, it is necessary to recognize at the outset that, in this case, the processes of assessment and management will probably be more complex and time-consuming than usual. A trainee who accepts this as a challenge rather than a chore, stands to gain a great deal of useful experience which has educational value when fed back to the management of the generality of patients. It also provides an opportunity for broadening of outlook and, perhaps, a chance to face up to some personal prejudices (from which no human being is immune).

The essential principle is that every patient must be viewed in the context of his or her particular social and cultural environment. Beliefs and behaviour must be assessed not against one's own norms but against those of the patient's own group. To this extent, transcultural psychiatry is simply good psychiatric practice.

HISTORY-TAKING AND EXAMINATION

Bear in mind that the diagnostic difficulties encountered, particularly where there is a language problem, may also have influenced the general practitioner or referring agent. They may have misunderstood the situation. Perhaps this is not a psychiatric case at all. The 'abnormal' behaviour may be simply an expression of grief, anger, or anxiety, in which case heavy-handed professional intervention, however well intentioned, could make matters worse: or organic illness may have been missed because the description of symptoms was misinterpreted. A careful physical examination should usually be done fairly early. Certain disorders, including anaemia, osteomalacia and tuberculosis (including tuberculous meningitis) are slightly more prevalent in ethnic minorities.

As soon as possible a collateral history should be obtained from a suitable informant, who can describe the sequential development of the disorder, confirm the precise nature of the symptoms, comment on the cultural normality or deviance of the behaviour or beliefs, describe the premorbid personality, and perhaps identify particular stress factors. It is often helpful to obtain this from more than one informant independently.

Interpreters

Where language is a problem the services of an interpreter must be obtained. In a crisis, or when some decisive intervention (e.g. compulsory hospital admission) is being considered, this is a matter of urgency. Remember that any relative or friend who accompanies the patient is probably not detached or impartial, unlikely to be a professional linguist, and certainly not trained in mental state assessment. *Under no circumstances should children be employed as interpreters.* Ideally every hospital and every social services office should have a list of interpreters on call for every language. They should have a contract with the authority and be paid. To obtain an interpreter ought to be no more difficult than to obtain emergency physiotherapy or an out-of-hours laboratory investigation when it is required for diagnosis or treatment. This is a counsel of perfection; in practice most authorities now keep lists of some sort because under the 1983 Mental Health Act there are statutory obligations on approved social workers to interview "in a suitable manner", and on hospital managers to ensure that the rights of detained patients are explained to them and understood. It is sometimes necessary to remind hospital administrators of this responsibility.

When working with an interpreter, remember that the interview will take longer than usual – in fact more than twice as long. It cannot be hurried. Before you begin, if you have not previously worked with that interpreter, have a private conversation and try to discover:

- What is the interpreter's training and previous experience in this kind of work?
- What degree of fluency does he/she possess? (A Hindi speaker may say they can "manage" in Gujerati, Punjabi or Bengali. A Cantonese speaker may not be adequate for all Vietnamese.)
- Does the interpreter have any personal or social contact with the patient's family?
- Does he/she understand about medical confidentiality?

You should then discuss the kind of information which will be sought in the interview and any difficulties you anticipate, e.g. with an angry or paranoid patient, or regarding particular symptoms (e.g. psychotic thought disorder). As a result of this preliminary discussion, it should become apparent whether the interpreter expects to be used as a linguistic technician, giving a word-for-word translation, or can do more than that. Experienced interpreters are able to use their own discretion in translating the meaning of questions and answers in a manner which is less precise, but may be more appropriate, and should be permitted to do so. This preliminary discussion should take place without the patient. The interpreter should also be given an opportunity to talk to the patient for a few minutes privately for introduction and reassurance. Ask the interpreter to check the patient's proper names for recording purposes, and to find out how he or she wishes to be addressed.

At the interview, the interpreter should sit next to the patient, to be 'on his side'. Address your questions directly to the patient and avoid having prolonged conversations in English in the patient's presence – take up points of detail afterwards. Remember that two of you (doctor and patient) are involved in the conversation only half of the time, but the interpreter is working very hard throughout without any opportunity to relax. Try to maintain eye contact with the patient, but do not be surprised if the main eye contact is between patient and interpreter. Utilize non-verbal cues; never display impatience or boredom; and be patient when a simple enquiry seems to lead to a protracted exchange, but be alert to the possibility that the interpreter may interpose his or her own opinions or advice, and discourage this. If necessary, terminate the interview and get another interpreter. With that exception, try to work with the same interpreter on all occasions. After each interview, allow time for feedback between you and the interpreter.

Despite the greatest care and thought, psychiatric diagnosis through an interpreter is usually unsatisfactory and diagnostic precision is always impaired. It is much better to arrange for the patient to be interviewed in his or her own language by a qualified person (e.g. doctor, nurse, social worker) who can not only translate but also participate in professional decision-making. This may not be possible immediately. It depends on a network of professional contacts or the existence of a multilingual team. In such a team the member(s) with the particular language becomes the therapist or 'key worker' for that patient, irrespective of discipline. Some non-English patients, however, show a tendency to overvalue doctors and undervalue other professionals, including nurses, perpetuating an unwanted class distinction which can be abrasive and may need to be worked through in team discussions.

Uncooperative patients

Especially where language is a problem, but in other situations also, remember that the patient may not understand the purpose of the interview and may not automatically assume that your intentions are friendly and helpful. Examples include the black person who has experienced racist oppression and victimization by white authority figures, and has come to believe that all white people are hostile; or a person who is in dispute with his or her family and thinks the hospital is a place for punishment; or a refugee who has experienced hostile interrogations, even torture, in the past. Fears which seem paranoid are not necessarily evidence of psychosis. A patient may be resentful or in a state of panic *because* of the psychiatric interview. It is often reassuring to permit a spouse or friend to remain in the room (English ideas about privacy and confidentiality are not shared by all cultures). If, however, there is any suspicion that the symptoms are a reflection of interpersonal problems, a strategy must be found for interviewing each one privately, possibly by involving a nurse or other colleague.

Physical examination

Standards of modesty and decency are different in Eastern cultures, and in general such patients should be examined by a doctor of the same sex. If this is impossible, a woman's husband should be allowed to stay with her when she is examined. Postponement of full physical examination may sometimes be the lesser evil. ECG and X-ray examinations are permissible and often reassuring. When arranging laboratory blood tests, remember that some patients do not know that blood is regenerated: they think that what is taken has gone for ever and its loss will cause permanent weakness.

Fear and stigma

In most other countries, insanity carries an even greater stigma than it does in Britain and mental hospitals are places of last resort. In many cultures the taint of insanity stigmatizes the whole family, and concealment or denial sometimes stands in the way of treatment. Hospital admission may be resisted, and a domiciliary visit preferred to an out-patient appointment. There may be reluctance to discuss interpersonal or family conflicts because it is shameful to reveal these to an outsider. Repeated reassurances about confidentiality may be necessary. Be prepared for important information to be withheld until the second or a subsequent interview.

Where hospital admission seems to be indicated, the reasons should be discussed with the patient and also with the family, who must be given an opportunity to suggest alternatives. It may be necessary to accept an element of increased risk and allow the patient to remain at home with frequent out-patient visits and support from a community nurse or social worker, but the risk must always be clearly stated to the relatives.

It is very seldom right to insist on admission against strong family objections. An exception is when the patient has run away from home to seek sanctuary because of maltreatment or denial of rights (e.g. an unwanted arranged marriage, or being taken out of the country). If this is suspected it might be right to provide temporary sanctuary, and even to deny access by relatives. The advice of social services should be sought: there may be a women's refuge or other facility which can provide an asylum more appropriate than hospital.

Ethical and legal problems may arise in relation to illegal immigrants and visitors not eligible for free treatment under the NHS. Consultant advice should be sought, and the local Community Relations Council may be helpful.

Doctors do not have any contractual obligation to act as informants for the Home Office: we should try to arrange that a patient who requires treatment receives it, and leave political and administrative questions to others.

MANAGEMENT IN HOSPITAL

The bewilderment and anxiety which all patients experience when first admitted to an institution are intensified a thousandfold for patients from other cultures, so extra consideration and kindness are required from all concerned. If any staff seem unwilling to provide this, it is a matter which should be explored in a suitable staff meeting. Patients with linguistic or cultural differences may not understand hospital rules and conventions, they may misunderstand instructions and be unable to make known their wishes. All patients should be asked about their requirements for prayer and other religious observances. For many people of other faiths these are very important. Diet is particularly important to Muslims, Hindus and Orthodox Jews, and exact details of dietary needs should be noted and passed on to the hospital catering manager. He or she should take these requirements as seriously as for any other special diet (e.g. diabetic), and provide meals which are appetizing as well as nutritious. It is sometimes necessary to remind catering managers of this responsibility, and the support of the UMT or Unit Manager may be required.

A patient who speaks little English and has nobody in the ward with whom to communicate, cannot benefit from group therapy, occupational therapy, or the continuous informal psychotherapy and counselling which other patients get from nurses and fellow patients. For such a patient, therefore, most of the hours spent in a hospital ward are, literally, a waste of time. If the only treatment the patient recognizes is brief encounters with a succession of doctors, these points of contact become immensely important. Such a patient may engage in attention-seeking behaviour because 'acting out' is the only option when other communication is impossible.

Bewilderment and boredom should be mitigated by reducing the time spent in hospital as much as possible. A patient should not be asked to remain merely to await a ward round or the results of an investigation. It may be possible to bend the rules about visiting hours, or encourage visits home in the care of relatives when behaviour permits and there is, literally, nothing better for the patient to do.

DIAGNOSTIC PITFALLS

Apart from the 'culture-bound syndromes' which are rare, the same mental disorders exist in all cultures, but they vary in presentation and symptomatology. Depression and anxiety are often manifested entirely by somatic symptoms in patients from Asia, and to a lesser extent Africa and the West Indies. One of the most confusing differences, which can lead to damaging misdiagnosis, is the presence of 'schizophreniform' symptoms as a stress reaction. Even when the behaviour and complaints seem floridly psychotic and include some first rank symptoms of schizophrenia, they may be stress-induced. Attention should always be paid to recent life-events. These and other diagnostic pitfalls have been described in detail elsewhere.

TREATMENT

Pharmacology

There are individual differences in the metabolism of psychotropic drugs and therefore in their therapeutic and toxic effects and dose responsiveness, and there is some evidence that populations differ in this respect. Tricyclic antidepressants should be given in lower doses to Asian patients and what little data there is suggests that the same may apply to phenothiazines. It is a safe general rule to start with smaller doses than usual of all drugs. The delayed effect of, for example, antidepressants has to be explained carefully as it is not readily understood or accepted.

Psychotherapy

Meaningful psychotherapy or counselling is only possible if there is a reasonable level of understanding. If you cannot communicate with the patient the only option is to find someone who can. Such a person may be found within the hospital staff or through social services or a community group. Even when a patient speaks good English there may be obstacles to developing a therapeutic relationship; for example many black people believe that it is impossible for a white doctor to appreciate the stress of being black in a racially prejudiced society. They have become cynical, often with good reason. Racism is endemic in Britain, sometimes deliberate but often due to ignorance and insensitivity. We have a responsibility to recognize this and try to avoid action or attitudes which may perpetuate it. Gender differences may be another barrier: an Asian woman may have difficulty in confiding in a male therapist, and a man from a male-dominated society may find it hard to accept the authority of a woman doctor or nurse. In any of these situations it may be necessary for you to work indirectly, relying on a third party (possibly a lay-person or relative) to carry out therapy under your supervision. Handled carefully this can be a valuable two-way learning experience.

Every culture recognizes mental disorder, and each has sets of explanations and conceptual models. Sometimes these include supernatural or magical beliefs which a scientifically-trained doctor finds hard to accept. Remember, however, that a culturally valid explanation is an asset to the patient and the family if it de-mystifies what is happening and offers hope. Any explanation is more comforting than none. We do harm by denying the patient's own explanations if we cannot replace them by alternatives which are understood and accepted.

Family therapy

Frequent mention has been made of the patient's family. This is because for most members of other cultures, and

Asians in particular, family cohesion and interaction are very important aspects of life, more so than for many indigenous patients. It is seldom possible or right to treat such a patient in isolation or as an individual, so 'family therapy' is not one option among others, it is the norm. Time must be allocated for talking with relatives, and their role in the treatment programme must be acknowledged and made explicit. By working with a family you will gain understanding of the norms, values and structures of that culture, and become less likely to impose alien ideas (your own) where these are inappropriate.

Further reading

Burke AW, ed. (1984) Transcultural psychiatry: racism and mental illness. *International Journal of Social Psychiatry. 30th Anniversary Double Issue 30:* parts 1 and 2 (Spring 1984)

Cox J, ed. (1986) *Transcultural Psychiatry.* Beckenham: Croom Helm

Henley A (1979) *The Asian Patient in Hospital and at Home.* London: The King's Fund

Littlewood R and Lipsedge M (1982) *Aliens and Alienists.* Harmondsworth: Penguin

Rack PH (1982) *Race, Culture and Mental Disorder.* London/New York: Tavistock

16

Mental Health Law

Keith J. B. Rix

In addition to the laws which have been passed by Parliament – Statute Law – there is also the Common Law based on judgements in seven centuries or more of individual cases. The legality of the trainee's acts and omissions in the course of his work is judged and to be viewed in terms of both the Common Law and such statutes as the Mental Health Acts.

THE MENTAL HEALTH ACT 1983 AND THE MENTAL HEALTH (SCOTLAND) ACT 1984*

Definitions

Mental disorder is taken to mean "mental illness, arrested or incomplete development of mind, psychopathic disorder and any other disorder or disability of the mind". Mental illness is not defined in the Act but the Memorandum indicates that "its operational definition and usage is a matter for clinical judgement in each case". The terms "mental impairment" and "severe mental impairment" are defined: mental impairment means a state of arrested or incomplete development of mind (not amounting to severe mental impairment) which includes significant impairment of intelligence and social functioning and is associated with abnormally aggressive or seriously irresponsible conduct on the part of the person concerned. Severe mental impairment is the same as mental impairment except for the degree of impairment of intelligence which is severe. "Psychopathic disorder" is defined as a persistent disorder or disability of mind (whether or not including significant impairment of intelligence) which results in abnormally aggressive or seriously irresponsible

---

*The Scottish Act is similar to the England and Wales Act. References to sections of the Scottish Act and to significant differences are printed in italics.

conduct. There is no definition of "any other disorder or disability of mind".

The Act goes on to say that on their own "promiscuity or other immoral conduct, sexual deviancy or dependence on alcohol or drugs" cannot be regarded as mental disorders which imply that "a person may be dealt with under this Act". Such persons may receive assessment or care on a voluntary basis and these conditions may be present in people who otherwise meet the criteria for mental disorder. "Medical treatment" as interpreted in s.145 includes nursing and also includes care, habilitation and rehabilitation under medical supervision.

In s.1 mental disorder is taken to mean "mental illness or mental handicap". "Mental impairment" and "severe mental impairment", by implication varieties of "mental handicap", are defined as in the England and Wales Act. There is no definition of psychopathic disorder, as such, but, for admission under ss.17/18 "where the mental disorder from which he suffers is a persistent one manifested only by abnormally aggressive or seriously irresponsible conduct" ('Scottish psychopathic disorder'), there has to be an expectation that "(medical) treatment (in hospital) is likely to alleviate or prevent a deterioration".

Section 125 interprets "medical treatment" as including nursing and also care and training under medical supervision.

Admission for assessment

If a patient is suffering from a mental disorder of a nature or degree which warrants detention in hospital for assessment (which may be followed by treatment) for at least a limited period and he ought to be so detained in the interests of his own health or safety or with a view to the protection of other persons, two registered medical practitioners can recommend admission under s.2 and such admission can be effected if an approved social worker (ASW) or nearest relative makes the application. One of the recommendations has to be made by a doctor approved as having special experience in psychiatry ('section 12 approved') and one has to be made, if practicable, by a doctor previously acquainted with the patient. Junior trainees will not usually make the first recommendation because in general the second one cannot be made by another doctor on the staff of the same hospital and, since the second would have to be made by a section 12 approved doctor, it is unlikely that the patient's general practitioner will be section 12 approved. However, if the trainee had previous acquaintance with the patient he could make one recommendation provided that the second could be made either by a section 12 approved doctor from another hospital or by a section 12 approved general practitioner who does not necessarily know the patient.

In an emergency the trainee might make a single medical recommendation for admission for assessment under s.4 but, in completing the form, he has to indicate how long a delay would take place if the patient was to wait for admission under s.2, i.e. how long it would take to obtain the *two* medical recommendations. If the trainee already knows the patient this means indicating how long it would take to obtain the second recommendation from a section 12 approved general practitioner or section 12 approved doctor on the staff of another hospital. If he does not know the patient he has to indicate how long it would take to obtain one medical recommendation from a section 12 approved doctor on the staff of the hospital and one from the patient's own general practitioner. Since there will almost certainly be a section 12 approved doctor on-call (duty SR or duty consultant) the length of the delay will usually be determined by the availability of the patient's own general practitioner. Once the trainee has made his recommendation on the prescribed form he needs to have an ASW or nearest relative to make the application.

If the patient is admitted under s.4 it is important to realize that once admitted there are only 72 hours in which to comply with the provisions of s.2 and effect the patient's detention for up to the full period of twenty-eight days. If the admission takes place on a Friday preceding a Bank Holiday or even a Saturday preceding a combined Monday and Tuesday holiday the trainee will have to take steps to contact the doctor(s) who will be examining the patient with a view to making the other medical recommendation(s).

Admission for treatment

Trainees will not usually make recommendations for admission for treatment (s.3) but if patients so detained are under their care they should ensure that they can always easily locate the date upon which admission took place. Thus they will be able to remind the consultant when renewal has to be considered (within two months of the date upon which the authority for detention would otherwise cease) and remind him when either the patient's consent or a second opinion is required if a particular treatment is to be continued (three months after the treatment was started – see Consent to Treatment).

No distinction is made between admission for assessment and admission for treatment. The grounds for admission (ss.17/18) are the same as for England and Wales with two qualifications to the effect that treatment is likely to alleviate or prevent a deterioration in the patient's condition if the mental disorder is 'Scottish psychopathic disorder' or if it is "mental impairment". This 'treatability' clause does not apply to "severe mental impairment". The two medical recommendations cannot be used as the basis for an application unless the patient is described in each as suffering from the same form of mental disorder (i.e. illness or handicap). One of the medical practitioners must be 'approved' according to the provisions of s.20. The 'mental health officer' (MHO) replaces the 'approved social worker' as one of the possible applicants for admission. In an emergency (s.24) a patient can be admitted on the recommendation of a single medical practitioner but, if practicable, the consent of a relative or MHO should be obtained.

Patients already in hospital

In an emergency for patients already in hospital, the alternative to s.4 is s.5. Under its provisions a patient can be detained for up to 72 hours on the basis of a report to the hospital managers by the RMO or his nominated deputy pending an application under s.2 or s.3. In some hospitals the RMO may nominate a junior trainee to carry out this task and trainees should make sure they know what the local policy is, particularly before acting as duty psychiatrist. The nominated deputy has to use his own clinical judgement and not simply carry out the RMO's instructions. This section also provides for qualified psychiatric nurses to effect the detention of a patient for up to six hours if the RMO or his deputy is not immediately available. Thus if a trainee is consulted by a nurse concerning a patient who, in the nurse's opinion needs to be examined with a view to the RMO or his nominated deputy furnishing a report under this section and either the RMO or his deputy (who may be the trainee) is not immediately available to attend, the nurse should be advised to consider using his holding power.

The procedure for detention of patients already in hospital is the same as that for s.24. The nurse's 'holding power' is effective for up to two hours.

Leave of absence from hospital

The RMO can grant a detained patient leave of absence (s.17, *s.27*) which, according to some Commissioners, he should record in the case records indicating the time at which it starts and finishes. If it subsequently appears to the RMO that it is necessary to revoke the leave of absence and recall the patient in the interests of his health or safety or for the protection of other persons this can be effected without making recommendations for a fresh compulsory admission. Both hospital records and letters or summaries sent to general practitioners should indicate if a patient is on leave of absence and can be so recalled.

Visiting and examination of patients

Any registered medical practitioner authorized by or on behalf of the patient's nearest relative to advise the nearest relative as to the advisability of discharging the patient (s.24, *s.35(3)*) or authorized by or on behalf of the patient or other person who is entitled to apply for the patient's discharge by a Mental Health Review Tribunal (MHRT) (s.76) may at any reasonable time visit the patient, examine him in private and see the case records relating to the patient's detention or treatment. Trainees should ensure that the case records are in order.

Consent to treatment

Decisions concerning treatment which require consent and a second opinion (s.57, *s.97*) and treatment which requires consent or a second opinion (s.58, *s.98*) are going to be taken by the RMO rather than the trainee. However, where a second opinion is sought from a Mental Health Act Commission (MHAC) appointed doctor and he needs to consult other persons professionally concerned with the patient's medical treatment, the trainee should ensure that all the appropriate records are in order and readily available and the other persons to be consulted will be available.

For patients compulsorily detained under s.3, psychotropic medication cannot be given for more than three months without either the patient's consent (which must be certified by the RMO or a MHAC appointed doctor) or a certificate from a MHAC appointed doctor to the effect that either the patient cannot understand its nature, purpose and likely effects or has not consented to it but needs it to alleviate or prevent a deterioration of his condition (s.58(3), *s.98(3)*). In order that the point at which the consent certificate is required is not overlooked the trainee should write in the records the first occasion upon which the patient is administered any psychotropic drug. If the patient was initially detained under section 2, this point may be reached *before* the patient has been detained for three months under section 3. The psychiatric team should be warned in advance of the three month date so, if a MHAC appointed doctor has to be called, there is time for this to be arranged.

Where the MHAC appointed doctor is considering a plan of treatment about which his opinion is sought, it is particularly important that it should be described and easily located in the patient's records. Although the plan will be that of the consultant and usually based upon discussion with the psychiatric team, the trainee may be expected to write it in the records during the ward rounds.

If 'urgent treatment' is required, detained patients (except those detained under ss.5(2), 5(4), 35, 37(4), 135 and 136) may be treated without their consent according to the provisions of s.62. If a voluntary patient or a patient detained under one of the above sections needs urgent treatment there are common law rights and duties to treat the patient (see below). Section 62 exempts the following treatments from the consent to treatment provisions of s.57 *(s.97)* and s.58 *(s.98)*: any treatment a) which is immediately necessary to save the patient's life; b) which not being irreversible is immediately necessary to prevent a serious deterioration in his condition; c) which not being irreversible or hazardous is immediately necessary to alleviate serious suffering by the patient, or d) which not being irreversible or hazardous is immediately necessary and represents the minimum interference necessary to prevent the patient behaving violently or being a danger to himself or others.

Second opinions are provided by medical practitioners appointed by the Mental Welfare Commission (MWC). The provisions for urgent treatment do not apply to patients detained under ss.24, 25(2), 117 or 118 of this Act or 177 or 378 of the Criminal Procedure (Scotland) Act 1975.

Mental Health Review Tribunals

If a patient appeals to a Tribunal (ss.65–79) or his case is automatically reviewed by a Tribunal, the trainee should study carefully the form in which the RMO's report is prepared and ask to attend at least some Tribunals in order to see how they are conducted.

Appeals are to a sheriff (s.35) rather than a MHRT but the MWC (s.3) also has powers to review the cases of detained patients and recommend their discharge.

Mentally disordered persons found in private premises or public places

The police may bring a mentally disordered person removed from premises under a warrant (s.135, *s.117*) or found in a public place (s.136, *s.118*) to hospital as a place of safety for detention up to 72 hours. Section 136 *(s.118)* states that the purpose is for the patient to be examined, interviewed by an ASW and for any necessary arrangements to be made for his treatment or care. Trainees who see such a patient need to realize that their attendance upon such a patient will usually constitute an examination and, if the patient needs admission for assessment or treatment, the procedures for such under s.2 or s.3 *(s.18, s.24)* need to be carried out before the 72 hours have elapsed. A registered medical practitioner has to be present when a patient is removed from premises under s.135 *(s.117)* and requests for such attendance received by a duty psychiatrist should be passed as soon as possible to the on-call senior registrar or consultant.

Section 118 makes no reference to examination by a MHO.

THE COMMON LAW

Parliament has not always adopted the active statute-making role it does today and previously legal questions were decided mainly by reference to the Common Law which is based on a collection of judge-made decisions. The system of precedent, applying the legal principles laid down in earlier cases on the same or similar facts, is central to the British legal system.

A number of these common law principles have a direct bearing on the relationship between the doctor and his patient. It is a *trespass to the person,* and damages can be claimed if there is an intentional unjustifiable interference with another. Clearly many of the day-to-day activities of a doctor potentially come close to a trespass to the person and it is only the old common law *defences* of *consent* or *necessity* that prevent a routine matter like an injection from being a cause of legal action in the civil courts as well as, in extreme cases, a matter for the police.

Consent does not have to be in writing nor indeed expressed orally, since a patient may indicate his consent by the way in which he behaves towards the doctor, for example, when he rolls up his sleeve before an injection of a multivitamin preparation. However, consent is not 'real' unless based upon sufficient and correct information about the nature of the treatment, its intended purpose and likely effects (including probable side-effects), substantial (but not unlikely) risks and its alternatives; an ability to understand these; and unless it is freely given. Ultimately, the nature and extent of the information is a matter of professional judgement. It is becoming increasingly important not only to be certain that these elements are present, but to specifically document the information given, to record an opinion concerning the patient's mental capacity to consent if this might subsequently be questioned and, with some patients, to record the name of a witness who could testify to the fact that the patient did not consent under duresss.

Sections 56–58 *(ss.96–98)* directly address the point as to what treatment can be given to which patients in circumstances where their real consent cannot be obtained. However, for informal patients and those detained under ss.4, 5(2), 5(4), 37(4), 135 and 136 of the Act *(ss.24, 25(2), 117 or 118 of the Scottish Act or 177 or 378 of the Criminal Procedure (Scotland) Act 1975)* real consent is necessary. If that is not possible then, to avoid a theoretical (or even actual) action for assault or battery, the doctor will have to rely on another old common law defence – that of *necessity*. This covers situations where a doctor has to give emergency treatment to save the patient's life; to prevent a serious deterioration; to avoid serious harm being done to other persons. If this occurs the incident should be documented as fully as possible as soon as possible with the names of witnesses if any.

A difficulty arises with patients, particularly the mentally handicapped or demented, whose conditions do not satisfy the criteria for detention under the Mental Health Acts, and yet either they are not unwilling to receive treatment, but their passive (implied) consent cannot be regarded as 'real', or they actively refuse or resist treatment. The College has recommended that in the case of the 'passive acceptor' the doctor should consider consulting the nearest relative (or substitute), other appropriate professionals, and another consultant, although ultimate responsibility lies with the doctor himself. For the 'active refuser', where the common law defence of *necessity* does not apply, similar consultation is suggested along with obtaining an informal second opinion from the patient's general practitioner.

The Mental Health Acts do not apply to treatment for physical illness in mentally disordered patients – unless the physical condition is causing or contributing to a mental disorder. Therefore in treatment in these cases there will be no statutory defence but the doctor will have to rely on the common law defences of *consent* or *necessity*.

A further implication of the common law is the basic sanction of an action for *negligence* if a doctor has not exercised reasonable care and skill in the conduct of his patient's affairs. A doctor, like any other person who provides a skill or service to others, has a legal duty to take care and if, as a result of a breach of that duty, the patient has suffered damage, a writ alleging negligence might follow. The duty to take reasonable care goes beyond clinical acts and omissions. A doctor can be said to owe an extra special duty to his patient beyond the ward and if he sees that patient at the hospital gate about to throw himself under a car and does nothing he will certainly be in breach of his duty of care to that patient. A technical defence that, for example, he has not been nominated by the RMO to act for him under s.5(2) will not defeat a claim in the civil court alleging negligence.

The MHAC's Code of Practice is likely to contain guidance on consent to treatment in relation to circumstances which are not covered by the Mental Health Act itself.

Further reading

Buglass R (1983) *A Guide to the Mental Health Act 1983.* Edinburgh: Churchill Livingstone

Department of Health and Social Security (1983) *Mental Health Act 1983. Memorandum on Parts I to VI, VIII and X.* London: HMSO

Gostin L (1983) *A Practical Guide to Mental Health Law.* London: MIND, 22 Harley Street, London W1N 2ED

Hamilton JR (1983) *Consent to Treatment: Questions and Answers. The Mental Health Act 1983.* Smith, Kline and French Publications 2(6)

Royal College of Psychiatrists (1985). Consent to psychiatric treatment for informal patients: College advice to psychiatrists. Report of the working party on the Mental Health Act. *Bulletin of the Royal College of Psychiatrists 9:* 228–230

17

Preparing Reports

T. Kay

At some stage in his professional career the practising psychiatrist will be required to report on one of his cases to a court of law, whether or not he has a particular interest in forensic psychiatry. Reports may also be requested by coroners, by tribunals, by compensation boards, or by insurance companies. Civil courts frequently deal with cases where one person takes action against another, whereas in criminal courts the accused is prosecuted by the Crown. In criminal cases the report may be requested by the court itself (the Procurator Fiscal in Scotland) or by solicitors acting for the defence.

Most cases referred to a trainee psychiatrist will be criminal cases and will most often be for magistrates' courts. Such courts are considered lower courts where a judgement of the facts is decided by magistrates who are laymen and are advised by the clerk of the court – a qualified lawyer. A stipendiary magistrate sits alone and is legally qualified. Magistrates' courts have no jury, unlike crown courts which are presided over by a judge who guides the jury in matters of law. Crown courts usually request a report from a more experienced psychiatrist. Magistrates' courts have relatively limited power of trial and sentence but both courts may request medical reports.

The following guide concerns reports prepared in criminal cases, but many of the principles apply to reports prepared in other circumstances.

REASON FOR REQUESTING REPORTS

Reports from psychiatrists are requested by the courts for several reasons, including doubt as to the accused's fitness to plead, the bizarreness of the offence or unusual behaviour in court. The courts may be aware of an earlier psychiatric admission. The defence solicitor may ask for a report for the same reasons and also as part of the defence where the plea is not guilty, or for use in mitigation where the plea is guilty. The psychiatrist should know who is instructing him and the reason for the request.

THE EXAMINATION

Individuals remanded on bail can attend the normal out-patient clinic. On occasion the court may remand the person on bail for the specific purpose of obtaining a report or the accused may be remanded on bail with a condition of residence in hospital for assessment. In more serious cases the remand will be into custody where the examination will take place in a prison.

Under the Mental Health Act 1983 the court also has the power of remanding to hospital under s.35 (Remand for a report) or s.36 (Remand for treatment).* Following a report to court s.38 (Interim Hospital Order) may be used to establish whether or not continued hospital treatment is necessary. Sections 36 and 38 do not apply to the charge of murder.

It is good practice to obtain as much information as possible from solicitors, previous medical records and depositions prior to seeing the accused. It is also good practice to interview relatives or close friends who may be able to shed some light on the accused's personality and behaviour, though this may not always be possible.

At interview, the psychiatrist should introduce himself and explain the purpose of his visit. He should explain the fact that the report may be used in court and that the accused is not obliged to answer any questions, but that the psychiatrist is impartial. Some psychiatrists seek the accused's

---

*The equivalent powers of the Scottish courts are derived from the Criminal Procedure (Scotland) Act 1975 (ss.25, 330).

written consent to prepare and submit the report. A full psychiatric examination following a standard schema should then be carried out.

It is tempting to start with the alleged offence, especially if there has been publicity, but it is best to establish a good rapport before discussing what could be very embarrassing topics. In taking the history certain questions have special importance. For example, the history of epilepsy should be excluded, especially in crimes of violence. Separately from epilepsy the history of 'blackouts' should be elicited as this is sometimes a defence. A history of venereal disease may suggest a personality disorder or may indicate a delusional belief in a psychiatric illness, and if the accused has not received treatment may raise the need for serological tests. In the case of a woman the menstrual history should be requested and premenstrual tension, if present, noted. In both sexes enquiries should be made regarding the individual's alcohol and drug consumption, as many offences occur in an intoxicated state.

The psychiatric history should include any present medication and the length of previous hospital confinement. The family history may suggest a sub-culture of criminality and in offenders there is frequently a history of a deprived background. Birth history, early development and childhood neurotic traits should be elicited.

Questions concerning educational achievements should be asked and should include truancy. The accused's ambition on leaving school may also be helpful as this, in conjunction with his employment record, may indicate a deterioration suggestive of a schizophrenic illness. The psychosexual development is of course important in sexual offences, and gives an indication of the accused's ability to relate well to another person. The health of his wife and children may point to family stress which could lead to crime. The personal habits and hobbies of the accused may suggest the presence or absence of a personality disorder where a rich appetite for drugs, alcohol and gambling may be present. The accused should be asked to give his own assessment of his personality including his ability to relate to others. Many highly dangerous men do not see themselves as dangerous.

PREVIOUS CONVICTIONS

In eliciting previous convictions the psychiatrist must be wary as the accused may genuinely forget to mention certain offences or may not wish to disclose them. The history should be checked with the police antecedant records. It is helpful to ask when the accused was first in trouble with the police, then to systematically enquire regarding Approved School, Youth Custody Centre, Detention Centre, Probation, suspended sentences, Community Service Orders and prison sentences. He should be asked if he has successfully completed any form of licence or parole. The specific nature of each offence should be recorded and the length of imprisonment should be recorded as the length of imprisonment will indicate the perceived seriousness of each crime. This information will allow the psychiatrist to see if the offences follow a pattern, e.g. committed when intoxicated or whether there is an escalating seriousness to the offences.

THE ALLEGED OFFENCE

The psychiatrist should train himself to always refer to the *alleged offence* and not the *offence,* even if the person says he intends to plead guilty. If the accused does not wish to talk about the offence or claims he cannot remember, then it is often useful to ask him what the police said he did or what others have told him. The events leading to his arrest may go back a considerable time and this should be borne in mind. The accused's activities on the day in question should be closely examined and if this includes use of alcohol or drugs the amount taken on the night before and throughout the whole of that day should be discussed. It should be asked if the person had taken meals during the day because of the possibility of hypoglycaemia or rapid alcohol absorption. In discussing details of the alleged offence when alcohol has been taken, the doctor should ask himself whether the person was too intoxicated to form an intent to commit a crime, but if the person describes an intent to carry out another act in immediate juxtaposition to the alleged offence, he will be deemed to have been capable of forming an intent to commit the alleged offence. Similarly the psychiatrist should assure himself that the accused was not in a psychotic state as a result of alcohol.

Claims of amnesia should be considered in the light of possible head injuries, severe intoxication or as a possible escape mechanism. However, it is not unusual for a person having inflicted many wounds, to remember only the first two or three wounds, whilst acknowledging responsibility for the others.

At the end of the interview the accused should be asked if he was properly cautioned by the police and whether he was properly treated by the police, given refreshments and periods of rest during interrogations. Specific complaints of threats of violence or permanent imprisonment should be noted and the doctor should consider the possibility of statements being made under duress and whether the accused had a vulnerable or suggestible personality. The *Judges' Rules on Interrogation and Taking Statements by Police* provide for the presence of a third party (e.g. a social worker) for a mentally handicapped child and a Home Office circular (109/1976) advises similar provision for mentally handicapped adults. This is not to imply malpractice on the part of the police, but occasionally statements are retracted on the grounds of duress or excluded by a judge if there has been a breach of 'Judges' Rules' or the circular guidelines.

Specific issues to be addressed in the examination include:

- Fitness to plead; that is he understands the charge, he can distinguish between pleas of 'guilty' and 'not guilty', he can instruct his legal representatives, he can follow the *evidence* and he can challenge a juror. Some judges may require that the accused can follow the court *proceedings* in general as well as the *evidence* in particular.

- His present mental state, particularly the presence or absence of psychotic illness, together with an assessment of cognitive functions.
- Mental responsibility for the alleged offence. This can be very difficult for the psychiatrist to assess and dogmatic statements should not be made. It may be that the psychiatrist can offer little help and the psychiatrist should be prepared to say so.

If possible, a link should be sought between the illness and the alleged offence and it is a useful exercise when offering a reasonable psychiatric explanation for the offence to then consider the most improbable explanation which may well form the basis of the legal adversary's argument. At this stage the treatability of the person should be considered and under what conditions that treatment, if any, should take place. This may range from out-patient treatment to treatment in a psychiatric hospital which may require the high security of a special hospital.

Physical examination should be carried out with reference to physical signs which may have psychiatric significance, e.g. liver disease, alcoholic neuropathy or evidence of drug abuse (see Chapter 7). Any scratches, bruises or bite marks should be noted that would support or refute alleged ill-treatment. However, the accused may have been in custody for a considerable length of time hence marks may have faded.

Deformities which would make the offence impossible or very difficult should be considered, such as abnormality of the hands.

With a psychiatric history and the physical examination complete, the doctor should consider the need for further investigations, such as blood tests, EEG, CAT scan, X-rays or psychological testing.

THE REPORT

Writing reports can be likened to pastry making. Both endeavours share a list of basic ingredients which vary slightly. For the trainee they also commonly fail to rise to expectations as in all matters practice makes perfect. The essential ingredients of a court report are:

- *Accuracy* – this is limited by the information provided. Particular care should be taken when the only informant is the accused. It should be remembered the report may be read out in court and it may be shown to the accused or to the parents of a juvenile. It should be written as the basis of possible examination and cross-examination in court and therefore the doctor should be able to answer for all the contents of the report. When accuracy is reliant on information from others, this should be indicated in the report.
- *Impartiality* – the report should be impartial as the psychiatrist's opinion is to assist the court by his specialist knowledge. However, impartiality is sometimes difficult to achieve when large fees are involved.
- *Simplicity* – it should be borne in mind that those making the decisions, namely juries and lawyers, have no psychiatric training and therefore technical terms and jargon should be avoided or explained; for example, electroencephalogram – brain wave test, delusions – fixed unshakeable false beliefs. Abbreviations such as 'pub' should be avoided and so should slang unless in inverted commas. Great care should be taken in using the words 'never' or 'always'.
- *Separate facts from hearsay* – try to corroborate the facts. Unconfirmed items reported by the defendant should be prefixed by "he told me" or "the accused said" and the source of unconfirmed hearsay should be indicated.

The report should be set out to show the basis for the opinions formed and the recommendations so that the reader follows a logical sequence which justifies the recommendations at the end, i.e.:

1. Introduction
2. The history
3. Previous offences
4. The alleged offence
5. The mental state
6. Opinion
7. Recommendations

Introduction

The report should give the person's name and date of birth and should commence by saying "I interviewed the above named at the request of" giving the source of the request and, if possible, the purpose of the examination. It should state when and where and how often the individual was interviewed and whether or not others were present. Some psychiatrists include the duration of the interview and if this is not given it is wise to know the length of the interview. The names of the informants and the source of all documents should be mentioned and the names of professional colleagues with whom the case has been discussed should be given. If any documents were not seen this fact should be reported. The depositions have special significance as their contents are considered to be true.

The history

The accused's standard psychiatric history should then be given. It is not necessary to mention a list of negative findings as the court will not be over-excited to learn of the excellent bladder functions of a young armed bank robber. Significant negatives should be mentioned. For example, it should be said that the accused specifically denied epilepsy or it may be recorded he had never seen a psychiatrist in the past nor felt the need to do so. Symptoms such as insomnia, constipation, lack of sex drive, or absence of menstrual periods could obviously support a diagnosis of a depressive disorder to be mentioned later in the report.

Previous offences and alleged offence(s)

Finally after giving details of earlier offences, the details relating to the alleged offence should be given. It is not the task of the medical practitioner to make the accused's situation worse and details which show him in a bad light should not be included unless it is for the specific purpose of indicating a degree of mental disorder which would require treatment.

Opinion

This should commence with the words "In my opinion" followed by a carefully worded statement outlining the elements of the history, his mental and physical state and the facts which led to the opinion reached. If other facts corroborate this information, these facts should also be mentioned. The nature of any mental disorder should be stated with particular reference to the categories employed in the appropriate Mental Health Act. The report should include a statement of the defendant's fitness to plead but it should be remembered that the decision in this matter is for a jury on the day of the trial and the doctor should be willing to express an opinion verbally to be heard by a specially empanelled jury. If the defendant is unfit to plead he will be sent to a place of safety and then to such a hospital as may be directed by the Secretary of State. If he is fit to plead then the information given should be such that if he is found guilty the court is clear whether or not he requires treatment by a psychiatrist and if so under what conditions. Reference should be made to prognosis, if possible, and with particular reference to dangerousness.

Recommendation

If a hospital order is recommended then the appropriate section of the Mental Health Act should be quoted and the completed section forms should be attached to the report. These require the doctor to state whether a bed is available and should indicate that the hospital concerned is willing to accept the patient. It is bad practice to recommend treatment but indicate that this should be under the care of another doctor in another hospital unless the doctor has specifically agreed. Although not commonly used, guardianship can be more suitable than hospital admission.

The court cannot insist upon a hospital admission without agreement from the doctor concerned or the managers of the hospital, nor may it impose conditions under which a patient can be treated within the boundaries of the hospital. However, a judge can make a condition such as 'security *a proviso*' in agreeing to a Court Order. The doctor must then consider whether he is willing to abide by these conditions in order to help the accused into hospital. The court may ignore the doctor's recommendations, there being good reasons to refuse a hospital admission. The recommendation will carry more weight if it also meets the dictates of common sense. Thus the psychiatrist will be unwise to recommend treatment in a hospital for serious violent crimes or sexual crimes if there is a chance that they may be repeated. Repetitive arson or severe child abuse could preclude hospital treatment and the psychiatrist's opinion should clearly indicate that he has considered the risk to the general public as well as the safety of the person concerned. The degree of security necessary should be a matter of paramount importance. It is impressive when the report can state that transfer to hospital is in the interests of the accused and *also* in the interest of the public at large.

It should be remembered that the s.38 interim hospital order cannot be used unless the accused is found guilty; this usually applies to s.37 hospital orders as well *(ss. 175 or 376 of the Criminal Procedure (Scotland) Act 1975)*, although a lower court can impose such an order without recording conviction or guilt if it is satisfied that the accused did the act or made the omission alleged. The two special verdicts of insanity ('McNaghten Madness') and unfitness to plead (insanity in bar of trial in Scotland) mean the patient has not been found guilty and must be dealt with under the Criminal Procedure (Insanity) Act 1964 or the Criminal Procedure (Scotland) Act 1975.

If the recommendation is for a probation order with a requirement of psychiatric treatment, the report should indicate the name of the psychiatrist by whom, or under whose direction, treatment will be given, whether treatment will be on an in-patient, out-patient or other basis, and where the treatment will be given. It is not necessary, although it may be helpful, to specify the nature of the treatment. It is good practice to liaise with the probation officer, who will have prepared a social enquiry report.

RELATIONS TO THE COURT

The doctor should realize that the court will regard his evidence as very important, but it may still only be a small part of the evidence used in the trial. There may be witnesses who would prove conclusively that the history given to the psychiatrist was wrong. It is salutary to remember that although a doctor has a right to have his opinion heard he does not have the right necessarily to have it believed or his recommendation acted upon. There may be overwhelming reasons why his opinions and recommendations are not practicable. The psychiatrist should not try to usurp the powers and rights of the court or to prolong the issue. Recommendations should not be outside the powers of the court. For example, magistrates' courts cannot impose a Restriction Order, not should there be vagueness about which hospital is concerned and when the bed will be available.

Remember, many intelligent laymen, including some lawyers, believe schizophrenia means Jekyll and Hyde, believe that we all suffer from depression, neurosis is a sign of weakness and epileptics are always violent. Many people believe that psychiatry has no place in a court of law and that most psychiatrists are themselves mad. The psychiatrist's report, therefore, should be evidence that the psychiatrist is a reponsible member of the public and not a specialist in a sympathetic but inept profession.

Further reading

Bluglass R (1979) The psychiatric court report. *Medicine, Science and the Law 19:* 121–129

Chiswick D (1985) Use and abuse of psychiatric testimony. *British Medical Journal 290:* 975–977

Gibbens TCN (1974) Preparing psychiatric court reports. *British Journal of Hospital Medicine 12:* 278–283

Grounds A (1985) The psychiatrist in court. *British Journal of Hospital Medicine 34:* 55–58

Haward LRC (1981) *Forensic Psychology.* London: Batsford Academic & Educational Ltd

Hoggett B (1984) *Mental Health Law, 2nd edition.* London: Sweet & Maxwell

Kenny A (1984) The psychiatric expert in court. *Psychological Medicine 14:* 291–302

d'Orbán PT (1986) Drugs and alcohol: the psychiatrist as expert witness in court. *British Journal of Addiction 81:* 631–639

Trick KLK and Tennent TG (1981) *Forensic Psychiatry (an introductory text).* Marshfield, Massachusetts: Pitman Publishing Inc

— 18 —
Studying and Examinations

Keith J. B. Rix

Professional training in psychiatry comprises clinical experience in appropriate training posts (see Chapter 1) and academic training for which arrangements vary from place to place. This chapter will describe both formal and informal aspects of the academic training in psychiatry and conclude with some advice concerning examinations.

STUDYING

The psychiatric tutor

The key role in co-ordinating some of the more formal aspects of academic training is undertaken by the psychiatric tutor (see Chapter 1). New trainees should see him at as early an opportunity as possible to find out about the local teaching arrangements.

Inceptorship of the Royal College of Psychiatrists

Upon the recommendation of their consultant, trainees may be admitted as 'inceptors' of the Royal College of Psychiatrists. They receive the *British Journal of Psychiatry*, details of College publications and notices of the national scientific meetings of the College and its Regional Divisions. The College structure also allows trainees to participate in various committees (see Chapter 19).

Day release schemes

Most SHOs and registrars use their study leave entitlement for day release courses run by their psychiatric tutor or local university department of psychiatry which prepare them for the MRCPsych examinations.

Some universities run Master's degree courses in psychiatry. These enable more able trainees to study for the MRCPsych and a Master's degree in parallel. Some of the university examinations are good practice for the equivalent MRCPsych examinations. Universities running such courses are Edinburgh (MPhil), Leeds (MMedSc), London (Institute of Psychiatry) (MPhil) and Manchester (MSc). The courses vary slightly in terms of academic and clinical content, examination arrangements and the dissertation. The University of Liverpool awards the degree of Master of Psychological Medicine to post-Membership trainees submitting an appropriate dissertation. This may soon become a taught course open to pre-Membership trainees.

Provided the trainee is on an approved training scheme and undertakes to remain in the scheme for the basic three years of the degree course, it is usual for the trainee's health authority to pay the course fees. Students who fail the class examinations or assessments may be allowed to attend the course as attached students in order to prepare for the MRCPsych examinations.

Residential courses

Short, residential courses of a few days are held in various places, but are best used for revision. They are no substitute for a course of study extending over months or years. They are usually advertised in the *BMJ* and *Lancet*. Trainees who have used all their study leave on day release courses may find it difficult to obtain paid leave to attend such courses.

The trainee's personal library

To begin with most trainees will want to acquire a textbook of general psychiatry, a textbook of descriptive psychopathology and a textbook about psychiatric emergencies. The choice of a textbook is difficult but most are likely to choose from those written by some of the leading British university departments of psychiatry. Subsequently books will be acquired according to the trainee's personal interests and according to the recommendations of teachers.

As an inceptor the trainee will receive the *British Journal of Psychiatry* but even the trainee who is not an aspiring academic psychiatrist would find a subscription to *Psychological Medicine*, the world's leading psychiatry journal, a valuable investment. *The British Journal of Hospital Medicine* frequently contains first-rate review articles of psychiatric interest and *Hospital Update* does so less frequently.

The trainee should also be constantly looking out for good review articles and key papers on various aspects of psychiatry and building up a comprehensive library of summaries, photocopies and reprints. The College publishes reading lists of key papers.

Filing systems

Papers and summaries or abstracts of papers need to be well organized and indexed. Trainees may be tempted to get by with just a dozen or more folders labelled 'Neurosis', 'Organic States' etc., but it may not be easy to locate what is needed. Most trainees need and deserve a better system.

First it is good discipline to make out an index card for every paper owned or abstracted and many papers which have been read and no more. If the abstract is brief, it can be written on the card, or if it is filed separately or if the paper itself is in the trainee's possession, the card can indicate where it is filed. The reference on the card should be complete and conform to a recognized convention such as the Vancouver System (devised by the International Committee of Medical Journal Editors) which gives the correct form for various types of reference (e.g. journal article, chapter in book, etc.). Time spent writing out the reference in full can save hours spent searching for the original when later the complete title, a third author's name or end page number is required.

One index system in use is the 'edge-punched card co-ordinated system' (Figure 18.1). The numerical holes along the edge of the card are allocated to aspects of psychiatry (e.g. 'neurosis', 'psychiatric epidemiology', etc.). The holes which correspond to aspects covered in the reference are clipped so that they become notches. The A–Z holes can be used to notch the initial letters of the authors' names. It is then possible to select all the papers on a particular topic or topics or all the papers by particular authors by passing a rod through the appropriate holes and shaking the cards so that those notched at a particular number or letter drop out (Figure 18.2). The cards do not need to be kept in a particular order and small bundles can be separated for various purposes and then put back with the rest at a later date. However,

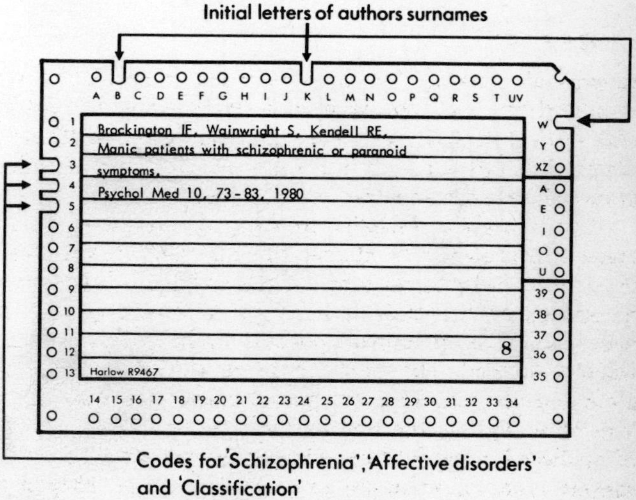

Fig. 18.1. Edge-punched index card

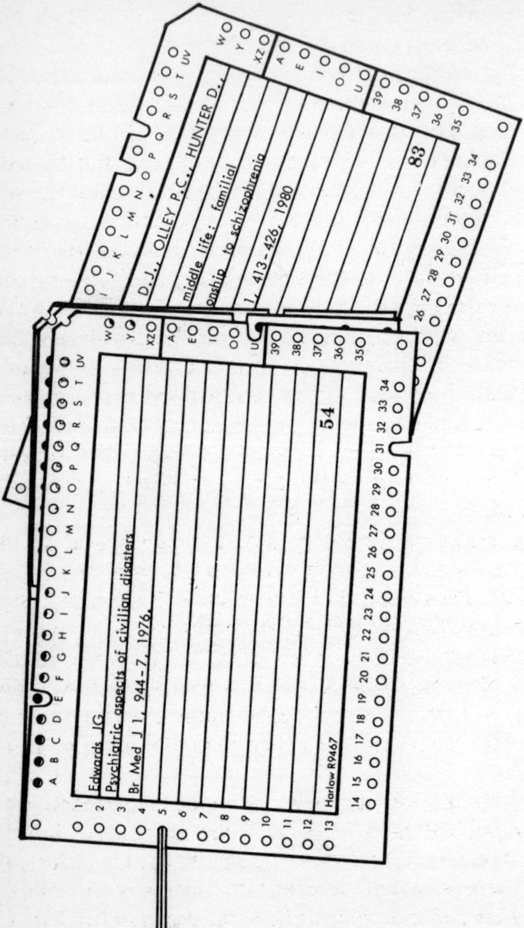

Fig. 18.2. Use of edge-punched card retrieval system

only a limited and relatively fixed number of aspects of psychiatry can be coded and the cards and rods are unwieldy if the number of cards exceeds about 150.

An alternative system, the 'accession number coordinated system', requires a separate but flexible index for the concepts or keywords by which references will be sought. Again each reference card bears an accession number by which the paper or reprint, if possessed, can be located but the accession number is also entered on every appropriate keyword card. Then from the alphabetically filed keyword index, the appropriate keyword cards can be used to obtain the accession numbers of all references covering a particular topic. According to the trainee's needs at the time he can go to the serially filed reference card, which may have an abstract or be eliminated from the search on the basis of the author or title, or he can go directly to the location of the actual reference. The reference cards have to be filed in numerical sequence, according to the accession number, since they are located by number.

The reference card may only indicate where information is to be found so the location of the reference should be specified. Thus, a further requirement is a system for storing reprints, photocopies and abstracts too long to write on the reference card itself. Unless the trainee has a small filing cabinet, the simplest method of storage is box files. Each paper or abstract has an accession number (which corresponds to that on the index card) and the papers are filed in numerical order.

Such index systems may soon be superseded by home computers, although at present the amount of information in a full reference to a paper is such that even modest numbers of references would exceed the memory of most home computers and searching a file for all papers with, for example, 'phobia', 'phobic' or 'agoraphobia' in the title would take too long.

Developing a library habit

Familiarity with the library includes a knowledge of its index system, knowing where the psychiatry, neurology, psychology and related books are to be found, knowing the location of current and bound journals, and knowing how to use *Index Medicus* and other aids to literature searching. Equally important is knowing how helpful the librarian can be *before* all else has failed.

The library should be visited regularly to survey systematically the current journals. For each journal the trainee might have a card upon which he crosses off the issue number after he has seen it (Figure 18.3). All trainees should make a point of looking at *Acta Psychiatrica Scandinavica*, the *American Journal of Psychiatry*, *Archives of General Psychiatry*, the *British Medical Journal*, the *Lancet* and *Psychological Medicine* at least.

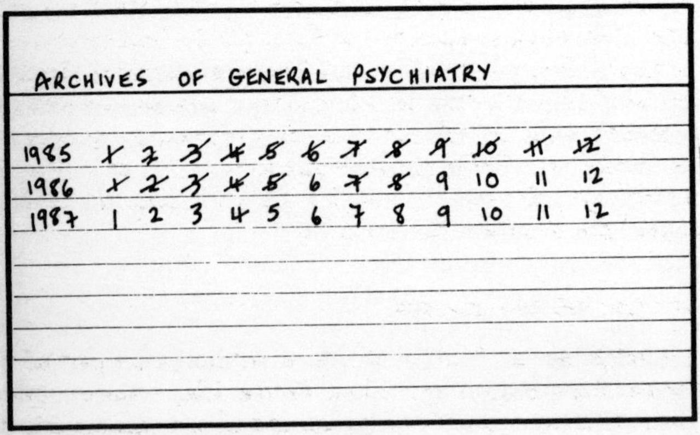

Fig. 18.3. Journal surveillance record card

Journal clubs

Most hospitals and psychiatric unit have journal clubs at which trainees present critical summaries of recent papers.

In some a blood sports flavour has been introduced and a good journal club is one in which the studies presented are mutilated beyond recognition. Such events do little more than call into question the corpus of psychiatric wisdom and put trainees off research. Choosing papers for journal clubs needs to be done carefully. Usually the best are ones with fairly robust methodology and something new to say. If you do not already have a journal club, get your psychiatric tutor to organize one and, if he does not do so, do it yourself. Trainees should take part in at least ten journal clubs a year.

Case conferences

You will be expected to attend at least 25 case conferences a year. Their format varies but usually a trainee presents a patient under the chairmanship of a consultant or other senior psychiatrist. Patients are chosen usually because they are difficult to understand, diagnose or treat. Occasionally cases are chosen because they are good illustrative cases.

Case conferences are useful for several reasons. Trainees get used to presenting cases to different consultants. In some places the case conference is regarded as practice for clinical examinations. There is the opportunity to hear different senior staff discuss some of the more complicated issues in psychiatric theory and practice.

The trainees' own records

Although, so far, 'case books' have not become a part of the formal examination procedure in the UK, trainees should keep their own records of typical as well as unusual patients. Some trainees keep copies of the case summaries or discharge letters of all patients who have been under their care. This may pose problems in terms of storage, security and confidentiality, but these problems are not insuperable.

THE MRCPSYCH EXAMINATION

Trainees who hope to go on to higher psychiatric training and obtain consultant appointments in the UK will not be appointed to SR posts unless they have passed the MRCPsych examination. The examination is in two parts.

Part I, usually taken after a year of psychiatric training, at present covers the neurosciences, including neuropharmacology, genetics, psychopathology and research methodology (including statistics and epidemiology). In 1987 most of the examination of these subjects will be moved to Part II and Part I will become an examination of interview techniques and basic clinical psychiatry. At present Part I comprises an MCQ paper and an essay paper. From 1987 it will comprise a clinical examination and an MCQ covering basic psychopathology (descriptive and dynamic), methods of clinical assessment in psychiatry, basic clinical psychopharmacology and some neuroanatomy, neurophysiology and neuropathology relevant to clinical neurology. The clinical examination will be concerned with basic clinical skills: the ability to relate to a patient, history-taking and mental state examination, and the exercise of judgement in bringing the relevant information together to make a succinct and accurate assessment. A detailed plan of management will not be required.

Part II is taken usually after three years of approved psychiatric training and success in Part I. It includes an MCQ paper covering aspects of general medicine applied to psychiatry, psychiatric disorders in children, adults and the aged, epidemiology relevant to psychiatry and the history of psychiatry. There is an essay paper with questions on general psychiatry, child psychiatry, mental handicap, forensic psychiatry and psychotherapy. From 1987 understanding of appropriate basic sciences will be examined in the essay and there will also be short answer questions. There is a clinical examination on a case drawn from any aspect of clinical psychiatry including mental handicap. General medical or neurological cases with a substantial psychiatric aspect may be included. There is also an oral examination.

Up-to-date rules and guidance can always be obtained from the College and it is particularly important to do so during the period over which the MRCPsych examination is being changed.

MCQ papers

The MCQ format presently used in the MRCPsych is the basic type in which an initial statement or stem is followed by a number of items or completions (usually five). Most questions include true and false items, but a question can contain all true or all false items. A counter-marking system is employed: a mark is given for each right answer and a mark deducted for each wrong answer. The purpose is to discourage random guessing. However, intelligent or informed guessing will usually result in more right than wrong answers.

Good technique requires a knowledge of the way certain standard terms are used. 'Typical' and 'characteristic' are used to refer to a feature which is of some diagnostic significance and in the absence of which the diagnosis might be questioned. A 'recognized' feature or effect is one that has been generally reported to occur and most candidates would be expected to know about it. The terms 'pathognomonic' and 'specific' refer to features which occur in the named condition but in no others. 'Majority' means more than 50 per cent.

There are a number of books of psychiatry MCQ questions. Trainees should practise with these.

In the exam the candidate should take note of the marking system. If it is counter-marking he should go through the paper answering only those questions about which he is fairly confident and which do not require a lot of thought. If he finds himself spending too long on a question he should leave it. The able candidate will get right questions answered the first time round. The second time round the candidate should try to work out the answers to those about which he has some knowledge. Again, he should get more right than wrong but the yield of marks will be less. The third time round the candidate should be cautious about answering the outstanding questions and avoid guessing. It is at this stage that some candidates may start to *lose* marks.

Usually answers have to be recorded on a separate sheet. Use this from the beginning, being careful to record answers boldly enough, otherwise on the next time round you may find yourself putting answers in wrong boxes. If all answers are put on the question sheet and transferred to the answer sheet at the end, mistakes may be made in transferring the answers.

Short answer questions

The new Part II examination will include short answer questions designed to test factual knowledge. Candidates will have to answer 20 questions in 90 minutes.

Essay papers

Some topics come up repeatedly so getting past papers from the College not only allows one to practise answering a particular question in a set time, but the trainee may have practised a question which crops up again, albeit in a slightly altered form. Careful study of recent review articles in leading journals may mean that the trainee is tapping the same source as those who set the questions.

It is important to read the instructions and the actual questions. If the instruction is '*Only* one question from Section A' there is no point in answering two. Reading the question is important for establishing what the examiner wants to know and what form the answer should take. There are always candidates who look for a key word (e.g. dementia) and then write down all they know about the topic. A discursive ramble is not 'a critical examination' or 'a discussion of the case for and against'. In general, essay questions are used to test the candidate's ability to communicate legibly and coherently, bringing together ideas and knowledge from a number of sources with a critical and balanced attitude. In the essay paper for the new Part II it will be particularly important to demonstrate the ability to integrate knowledge from the basic sciences with clinical aspects of psychiatry.

The clinical examination

Before the examination it is essential to have been through some mock examinations. Some tutors organize these but some trainees take it upon themselves to organize them, inviting local consultants to be mock examiners.

It is important to pay attention to appearance. Examiners are only human and they may be adversely influenced by candidates who are unclean, untidy, over-dressed or seductive. In most clinical examinations the candidate has an hour with the patient and five minutes to prepare his formulation. Most candidates would be advised to spend 30 to 40 minutes taking a brief history, 10 minutes completing the mental state examination and, if appropriate, covering some aspects of physical examination and 15 to 25 minutes working on the formulation (see Chapter 9). The candidate should ensure that the patient stays near at hand in case any point has been missed.

Preliminary questions can cover areas such as what the doctors say the diagnosis is, what investigations the patient has had and what treatment he has had or is going to have. If the patient is an unreliable, poor or difficult historian and particularly if this results, for example, from acute psychotic disturbance or a possible organic syndrome, the candidate may be advised to skim some aspects of the history, and concentrate on carrying out an impressive mental state examination.

In the Part II clinical the examiners will usually expect about a five minute summary ('assessment'*) of the salient

---

*The College does not use the term 'formulation'.

history and examination findings, with a discussion of diagnosis and differential diagnosis, and an account of supposed aetiology. The balance will depend on the type of patient and flexibility is advisable. Next it is usual for the candidate to be asked to interview the patient briefly in the presence of the examiners. After this the candidate is likely to be asked to discuss treatment (including a plan of investigation) and prognosis.

On meeting the examiners' time is at a premium. Slow, circumstantial or detailed answers leave less time for other questions and if one line of questioning reveals weaknesses, there may not be time for the candidate to redeem himself on other questions. Sometimes under exam conditions a candidate omits something important. Acknowledging this, rather than trying to hide the omission, makes a better impression and there may be the opportunity to expand upon the point in such a way as to indicate that one would usually enquire in this area and also demonstrate how one would use the information acquired.

The oral examination

In Part II the candidate sees a different pair of examiners for a 15 minute oral examination, but this will be 30 minutes from 1987. Much of what has been said about the clinical examination also applies. Here, if the candidate does not know the answer to a question, he should say so rather than waffle or shift the answer to a related topic. Examiners are more impressed by honest candidates who admit their shortcomings than by devious candidates who struggle, usually unsuccessfully, to hide them. Increasingly the questions in the oral examination are 'patient management problems' rather than theoretical questions.

Feedback

If a candidate fails he can write to the College Dean and ask for an account of his performance.

Further reading

De Alarcon R (1969) A personal medical reference index. *Lancet i:* 301–305

Eagles JM and Alexander DA (1987) *MCQ Examinations in Psychiatry.* Aberdeen: Aberdeen University Press

Farmer R (1984) *Self-assessment in Psychiatry.* Oxford: Blackwell

Gill PV and Spear FG (1986) A different reading list for MRCPsych? *Bulletin of the Royal College of Psychiatrists 10:* 284

International Committee of Medical Journal Editors (1982) Uniform requirements for manuscripts submitted to biomedical journals. *Annals of Internal Medicine 96:* 766–771

Morton LT (1978) *How to use a Medical Library, 6th edition.* London: Heinemann

Roberts DC (1984) The organization of personal index files. In Morton LT and Godbolt S, eds. *Information Sources in the Medical Sciences,* pp.512–522. London: Butterworth

Royal College of Psychiatrists (1984) *Rules for Entry to the Membership Examination (M.R.C.Psych.) Including the Preliminary Test.*

Royal College of Psychiatrists (1985) *Working Party for Review of the M.R.C.Psych. Report to the Court of Electors*

19
Committees

Tim Jerram

Committees are unpopular: they are the butt of many jokes, frequently regarded as time-wasting and are regarded as inferior to 'real' work such as seeing patients. Although also frustrating and boring, they are democratic and are often the only way of achieving certain tasks and anybody who plans a career in the Health Service, especially in the hospital service, will have to spend at least some time in committee work.

GENERAL

A committee can be defined as a group of people, usually established by an authority or an organization, who meet, under agreed procedures, to carry out certain tasks. These tasks may be of two sorts – the committee being either an 'advisory' or 'executive' one. Usually executive committees operate at a senior level (such as the Council of the College or a health authority) while more local committees (such as a division of psychiatry) are advisory. The distinction is often blurred – for instance a local division will have some executive functions – but is important. Similarly people become members of committees in various ways – because of their jobs, because they hold a particular post *(ex officio)* or because they are nominated or elected by other people. In the latter instances they are either 'representatives' (who 'represent' their sectional interests) or 'delegates' – regarded as sensible people who will make wise decisions on the evidence before them. This distinction is nicely reflected in the US Congress where each member of the House of Representatives has a similar size constituency whose interests he protects, whereas each state elects two members to the Upper House (Senate) which is then supposed to act independently for the overall good. Failure to appreciate this distinction can lead to embarrassing and unreal demands being made, for instance where a doctor is a member of a health authority.

Trainees are likely to become involved with a committee in one of three main areas:

- In the NHS there has to be some form of medical advisory machinery and usually this is in the form of divisions. Each division covers a major speciality or hospital (medicine, surgery, psychiatry, etc.) and should have one or more trainee members. Inevitably the division has to take on some executive functions which often affect trainces. They include such things as duty rotas, allocation of staff and use of facilities like out-patient or day hospital accommodation. It appoints the psychiatric tutor, advises on library facilities and (perhaps with one or more other divisions) sets up a committee to oversee a rotational training scheme. In addition, individual hospitals or units will have some form of medical staff committee including senior and junior staff: this would be the forum to bring problems to which cannot be resolved individually – poor on-call facilities, difficulties with the Pharmacy, procedures for admissions and so forth.

  Below this level there is likely to be a variety of committees or groups – covering, for instance, a small number of wards or a unit, an area of work such as rehabilitation or a users' committee of some facility like occupational therapy. They are usually informal, but can be a useful experience, especially in learning the arts of talking in committees and making compromises.
- The Royal College of Psychiatrists. Its central body is Council and trainees are represented there through the Collegiate Trainees Committee (CTC) which is a special committee of Council and to which it is responsible. CTC members sit on every College committee except the Court

of Electors. The CTC comprises 86 trainees elected from the regional divisions, four *ex officio* members (the Dean and three Sub-Deans of the College) and two co-opted members. There are four meetings a year coinciding with the College quarterly meetings and an additional residential meeting each September. The College itself has 10 regional divisions covering the whole of the British Isles. Each has an executive committee which organizes day meetings and meetings for trainees. Trainees in the division have at least two seats on this executive. Your psychiatric tutor should know who they are and how they are elected.

- There is a variety of other committees including joint ones with social services (especially planning for new facilities or client groups), advisory committees for hostels and voluntary groups and liaison with other professional and lay groups. Although these are often seen as good experience for trainees, the demands made may be rather different with the medical members being expected to act as 'expert witnesses' rather than ordinary committee people.

PROCEDURES

The constitution

This is normally written (somewhere!) but occasionally will have become accepted with the passage of time. It should at a minimum contain the following information:

- *Membership* – clearly spelled out, e.g. if "all consultants" are members, does this include those with part-time or honorary contracts? What about those in sub-specialties – child psychiatry and mental handicap or those whose beds are in another hospital? Other members may be defined by post title ("The Divisional Nursing Officer") or by a parent body ("One representative from the Division of Medicine"). In the latter case it is assumed that the sending body is responsible for ensuring that it is properly represented. Certain people may be identified as observers, non-voting or co-opted members.

- *Officers* – it should specify what officers are required. Usually there will be a chairman and secretary, but there may be a vice-chairman and a treasurer. Sometimes the duties of the secretary and minute-taker are divided (into correspondence and records secretaries). The constitution should specify whether these posts are open to all or are restricted to certain members (e.g. does the chairman have to be a consultant?).
- *Frequency of meetings* will be specified, e.g. "not less than four times a year": it will state when the Annual General Meeting (AGM) takes place.
- *Quorum* – a committee's decisions arc of little value if they arc taken by a very small group of people, so it will state what number (either relative or absolute) of members must be present.
- *Annual General Meeting* – this is an opportunity for the committee and its members to reflect on its workings; office-holders are elected or re-elected, membership of sub-committees is reviewed and any alterations made to the constitution. Rarely, when major or constitutional issues come up at other times (such as loss of confidence in the chairman) an Extraordinary General Meeting (EGM) is called.

Sub-committees

These are of two types, either permanent or temporary.

- Permanent sub-committees may be prescribed in the constitution. The most significant is some form of executive committee, though this may not be clear from its title. More commonly, the title such as "Executive" or "Finance and General Purposes" does reflect its role. For instance in the College, Council is a large, unwieldy body which meets quarterly: obviously this is insufficient to transact all the business and much of this is done by the Executive and Finance Committee. The discussions and decisions will be ratified by the full body. Otherwise most permanent sub-committees will be concerned with a specific task or area, e.g. the Library; future planning; out-patient accommodation, and so forth.

- A temporary sub-committee (also known as a working party, working group, *ad hoc* group) is set up to consider a specific topic – a Government proposal, the job description for a new post and so on. The important thing is that its terms of reference are clearly laid down and some indication is given of how long the task should take. Subsequently a report is presented outlining the reasons for setting up the group, the factors they took into consideration and their formal recommendations: these are then accepted or amended and the sub-committee discharged.

Agenda

The agenda is usually drawn up by the secretary and/or chairman. With a small or informal committee such as a division of psychiatry this is a straightforward matter, but larger committees, such as boards of medical schools, etc. may have an agenda sub-committee. In either case someone should ensure that matters brought forward to the committee are properly prepared (with background papers available and proposals clearly defined), that the agenda is not too long and that there is a reasonable balance between items. Important committees – regional health authorities, the Council of the College, district medical executives and so forth, which receive reports from many sub-committees and other bodies, can have very lengthy, formal agendas and specified items will only be discussed if an individual member wishes them to be or the officers consider it advisable.

The minutes

These are vital documents. At the very least they should record who was present; what items were discussed and in which order; what decisions were agreed and which motions, if any, were passed. Usually they will contain some account of the discussions that took place, especially of those views which were expressed very strongly.

The secretary, as soon as he can after the meeting, prepares a draft which the chairman reads. If he feels they are accurate they are then circulated to all members, usually with an agenda for the next meeting. At this the committee will be asked to approve them as a full and accurate recording of the deliberations. This not only allows minor errors to be corrected (titles, initials, names missing from the list of those present, typing errors), but also enables anybody who feels that the discussion or views stated have been ignored or misrepresented to correct them. He points out the error and suggests a phrase or sentence which can be added to, or replace part of, the minutes to make the meaning clear. This must not become an opportunity for people to re-open or continue the discussion, but it should be confined to the facts of what was actually said or done at the time. After this the chairman will ask formally if he can sign the minutes and do so. Particularly when a committee meets infrequently, the minutes may be circulated quite widely before this happens: although this is acceptable these minutes are then, as yet, unapproved. The secretary then preserves the signed copy in a complete and permanent record of the committee's meetings, which can be consulted by members, if and when necessary. Ultimately such documents may even become archival so should be treated with care.

Conventions

All committees operate within a series of conventions which govern behaviour and the conduct of business. At first sight these may be mystifying or even ridiculous, and the strictness with which they are followed depends on the formality and size of the committee, but even the most informal committees may have to fall back on them when controversial or difficult matters are being discussed. The main ones, however, are the following:

- *Conduct* – in a civilized committee only one person speaks at a time, and the chairman controls who is speaking, although a conversational style of business is quite common. In more formal committees the person speaking should only be interrupted on a "point of fact" or "information" (where the speaker appears to be making an error) or on a "point of order" (where the person is not following the conventions such as by deviating from the topic, repeating old arguments or making personal comments).
- *Chair* – all remarks are addressed to the chairman and indeed to the office rather than its holder, which explains why a committee member may be heard addressing an old friend (or even enemy) in the seemingly formal and archaic phrase "Mr Chairman".
- *Motions and resolutions* – ultimately any executive committee has to decide on a specific course of action and this is usually expressed in some formal way. If a clear consensus exists it may be adequate to record "It was AGREED that, etc. . ." but in more formal and important settings this will require that the committee accepts a motion. Such a motion is often available to members before a meeting or at least clearly stated at it ("tabling"). After debate, the motion (or resolution) is proposed and seconded formally by named members, or the chairman will call for someone to do this. Other members may suggest amendments to the motion which may modify it or even negate it entirely.
- *Voting* – committees with a purely advisory function will rarely vote. Executive ones will have to do so more frequently, but the rules are the same. Firstly the committee should be absolutely clear what it is voting on – hence the need for a clearly-drafted and easily understood motion. The vote may be taken in any form – a show of hands,

orally or a ballot – although the last is usually only needed for the election of office-holders. With formal motions, the amendments are voted on first; if they fall then the original motion is voted on. Most committees operate on a simple majority, unless the constitution specifies otherwise, and it is usually necessary to have a greater majority (e.g. "two-thirds of the membership") for a change in the constitution itself. If the vote is a tie the chairman usually has a casting vote *which is additional to the one he has as member of the committee.* Conventionally, this is used to maintain the status quo, although this is not invariable.

- *Loyalty* – once a decision has been properly and democratically made, all members of a committee should then stick by it ("doctrine of collective responsibility"). There are safeguards if you feel strongly about an issue – you can ask for your objection to be minuted, you can, if appropriate, enter a minority report or you can resign from the committee!

PRACTICAL ADVICE

Skills in committee work can be improved by studying those who are good at it and by practising. Trainees are often in an excellent position to do both, especially the former. Do try to be an office-holder of some sort, if only because appointments committees usually look for administrative experience.

The chairman

The chairman has duties both inside and outside the meeting. Prior to the meeting he will familiarize himself with the business, estimate which items are going to be controversial or lengthy and arrange with the secretary that they come at an appropriate place on the agenda. With complicated matters he will introduce the topic, summarizing the present situation before inviting opinions. He then has the task of controlling the discussion – preventing repetition and the discussion from becoming a dialogue, and encouraging the less strident members to contribute. At some stage he will decide when the topic has been adequately debated and then sum up, very briefly, the discussion so far and express the views of the committee. The timing of this calls for considerable skill. If he stops the discussion too soon some members may feel aggrieved that not all the points have been covered, and although there may be superficial agreement, the topic will probably crop up again or factions may develop outside the meeting. On the other hand, if the discussion goes on too long some people will become bored and take no part in the proceedings: others will become too involved and perhaps adopt extreme positions which they may subsequently regret. It can be instructive to compare chairmen and their degree of authoritarianism – obviously the one who has a clear idea of which decision he prefers and is fairly forceful about it is likely to get his way: this may not, however, lead to the best long-term solution. Occasionally it will become clear that no agreed decision is possible. If the committee is an executive one it will then be necessary for the issue to be voted on, but for an advisory committee the chairman will try to find a consensus view. If it is clear that there is none, the chair is best advised to defer discussion to a subsequent meeting, allowing members to reflect on the matter further and consider new arguments. For important issues he may suggest that a sub-committee be set up to work out a solution, so preventing the main committee getting bogged down on one issue.

The chair also has functions outside the meeting. He can make rapid decisions where necessary ("chairman's action") and represents the committee elsewhere. Informally he may give a view as to how his committee will react to a proposal.

The secretary

The secretary has two main duties – keeping the minutes and generally servicing the committee administratively:

- The minutes are the only permanent and ultimately legal record of any discussions. The sensible secretary will take copious notes during the meeting and should be absolutely clear of the wording of any formal motions or decisions agreed. It is better to clear up any doubts at the meeting than to say "we will sort it out when we write the minutes" as the secretary then either has to make the decisions himself or leave the minutes deliberately ambiguous which achieves nothing.
- This is a thankless, boring but vital set of tasks, without which no committee can function. The secretary is responsible for organizing the individual meetings – booking the room and refreshments, ensuring that an agenda is prepared and that appropriate papers are circulated in time for the meeting. He should give notice of the AGM and remind members of the nomination process, being prepared for any elections that ensue. Secondly, he is the correspondent of the committee: all correspondence should either emanate from him or he should receive a copy if others (e.g. the chairman) write letters and he should receive letters addressed to the committee, or copies of them. Thirdly, he retains copies of all minutes, documents and letters and files them appropriately. The minute book should be properly indexed (usually the items or topics are indexed alphabetically with a cumulative list of where they appear in the minutes).

Committees function best in proper surroundings (e.g. not the corner of the mess), when their tasks are clear (hence the need for a clear agenda), and by not going on too long (up to about 90 minutes, except for a very formal committee).

The ordinary committee member

When elected or put on a committee establish your role (representative or delegate?) and your rights (can you vote, for instance?). Spend one or two meetings getting to know how this committee works and ensuring that you know who your colleagues are and who they represent. Watch those people who seem to be listened to and try to work out why. Try also to pick up undercurrents – does Dr X always oppose Mr A's suggestions regardless? Does Dr Y always agree with the last speaker and so forth? Do not feel that you have to comment on each topic: if there is something about which you want to speak make sure that you are adequately briefed (e.g. reading a background paper or report, reminding yourself of some regulations or discussing it with colleagues you are representing). Have a clear idea of what you will say – jotting down headings or points and then enumerating them helps the secretary and means that what you say will be minuted accurately. After you have finished, note any questions or points made by other speakers – you may want to rebut them subsequently and it will also help you to report what happened to any interested parties, e.g. other trainees. When the minutes come round, check that they are correct in that they record what you said (which may not be the same as you think you said!). It is then quite easy to keep the issue alive by raising it under "matters arising" or asking for it to be put back on the agenda. Be prepared to lobby for your cause – pointing out to others the background to and advantages of your proposal – in between meetings. Committees tend to be conservative and often inert, so watch out for possible stalling techniques. These include suggesting that this committee is not the appropriate one to deal with the matter, referral to a sub-committee or a bland minute which promises no particular action.

Finally, do not become seduced by committeedom. Often the best chairmen and members are the reluctant ones who are also good at their other tasks. A committee is only ever a means to an end and its effectiveness should be judged solely on those ends.

Further reading

Chaplin NW (1982) *Health Care in the United Kingdom: Its Organization and Management.* London: Kluwer Medical
DHSS (1980) *Organizational and Management Problems of Mental Illness Hospitals (Report of a Working Group).* London: DHSS
Finch JD (1981) *Health Service Law.* London: Sweet and Maxwell
Hall L (1984) *Meetings: Their Law and Practice.* (Revised by Lawton P and Rigby ER.) Plymouth: McDonald and Evans
Martin JP (1984) *Hospitals in Trouble.* Oxford: Basil Blackwell
Scott J (1986) The functions of the Collegiate Trainees' Committee. *Bulletin of the Royal College of Psychiatrists 10:* 64

— 20 —

Planning Psychiatric Research

David Goldberg

"Research is to teaching as sin is to confession" is inscribed round the library of a seminary in St Louis – if you don't do any of the former, there is nothing to talk about in the latter. The situation is getting even worse than that for psychiatric trainees: such is the competition for SR jobs that the trainee who hasn't yet started on a project is likely to be at a severe disadvantage.

In your first year as a trainee you therefore have two tasks – to decide whether psychiatry is really for you, and to give serious thought to a research project. By the time you get your registrar appointment you should have started preliminary work, as there will soon hardly be enough time if you are to have something to put down on your SR application form in two or three years time.

GETTING STARTED

It is relatively easy to think of questions to which no-one knows the answer: the trick is to think of one that could be illuminated by a single person working in their spare time which hasn't been answered already.

Thinking of an idea yourself

Generally speaking, ideas for one-man projects will be suggested by a clinical problem that you have encountered, or by something that you have read in the library. In either case, you are more likely to elaborate on your ideas if you have a *notebook* in which you jot down ideas, and sugges- tions made to you by others about references that you might read. (Once you have got started, this same notebook will go up in the world, and will be called your *"project log"*, of which more later.)

It is very desirable to think of some project which can be incorporated into your usual working week: thus a project dealing with the effects of diagnosis on the occupational adjustment of first admissions could easily be done while you are doing any general psychiatry training post, whereas an epidemiological project which involved you interviewing a probability sample of the normal population would be very difficult to carry out in one's spare time. As soon as you think that you have an idea for a project, go to the library and read up whatever you can find about your chosen topic in, say, three visits to the library (see below). This should give you good ideas about the measuring instruments that you might use, and you will note the statistical procedures used by others engaged on similar projects. It is now time to discuss your ideas with someone more experienced: so, choose the person in your hospital with an interest in your chosen field, and ask for an appointment. (Try to choose someone who has a good publication record themselves: they will give you better advice.)

Asking someone else for a project

There is no shame in doing this: it is a very good way of getting started. Not everyone finds it easy to think up an original idea, but most trainees are able to carry out a project under supervision. However, you will need to have some idea of the general area in which you are interested, and you must be prepared to go away to a library and read round your assigned topic, so that you can impress your supervisor by making constructive suggestions of your own about further improvements to the project. Beginners are often attracted to psychotherapy research, but they should think twice unless they have very definite ideas of their own. It is probably the most difficult area of all in which to carry out a one-man project reasonably well, and it may be difficult to find a suitable supervisor.

USING THE LIBRARY

If you have got hold of a good recent paper on the subject of your choice, use the references at the back to find other papers: this is going backwards in time. If there is a classic paper that came out some years ago, look it up in the 'Citation Index' in order to go forwards in time. Alternatively you may be able to carry out a computer search on your chosen topic: most librarians will be pleased to advise you about appropriate 'keywords' to use in such a search.

COLLABORATING WITH OTHERS

It does not matter if you are part of a larger team on a project, providing that your dissertation clearly indicates how much work you carried out yourself on the project, and how much was done by others. In any publication, these other workers will of course appear on the title page, but it is usually possible to give a single worker a part of a large data-set to write up themselves as a Master's dissertation.

THE RESEARCH PROTOCOL

No research is worthwhile unless a question is formulated: the art is to pose a question that can be answered, and whose answer is not already known or self-evident. It is also helpful if the answer to your question matters. Although your protocol will start with this question, you should not try to frame the exact wording of the question until you have roughed out the method, decided on the measures, and carried out quite a lot of reading of your own.

The research protocol should be *refreshingly short, and easy for your supervisor to read.* This means that ideally it will fit onto a single sheet of A4 paper.

The protocol uses the following headings: title; aim; method; measures; ethical aspects; treatment of results.

It is essential to make proper notes of your reading, and to record the full reference of each paper in the form in which it may appear in your dissertation (see p.232). (Many people do this on cards.) However, you must resist the temptation of writing any of this on your research protocol: *it is simply not necessary.* Save it for the 'literature review' part of your dissertation!

Method

By this time you have a rough idea of what you actually intend to *do* – this is the **method**, so jot down some notes about this first. Where will the patients come from, and how many can you reasonably expect to assess in the time available? Is it possible to estimate the number of subjects that you will need, or will you need a pilot study?

Measures

Almost inevitably, you will be using some measuring instruments: perhaps a laboratory procedure, or a psychometric assessment like the Present State Examination. These are your **measures**, and they go down next. Sometimes you will need to invent a measure for a particular project: an example would be a trainee who devised a gadget so that patients with over-valued ideas about the size of their nose could indicate the size and shape of their perceived nose. Don't be too ambitious: remember that if you are producing a new measurement procedure this could itself be your entire project! Remember that measurements on some new measure must be related to something known – either another established measure, or to criterion groups of subjects.

Ethical aspects

If patients are to receive measures that would not normally be made, do you need ethical approval? You will certainly need ethical approval before blood can be taken or a drug can be randomly assigned: many hospital ethical committees now insist on vetting applications which merely subject patients to enquiries or psychological treatments which they would not otherwise have had. Ask if your local ethical committee uses a standard form, and get hold of one.

Treatment of results

The **treatment of results** heading serves as a reminder to you to answer three questions:

1. How will you collate the data?
   - Is there so much that it will have to be transferred to a mainframe computer? (If so, what programme will you use, who will pay expenses, are you going to learn to operate a terminal yourself?)
   - Will you do it yourself on your personal micro?
   - Is it feasible to enter it all on a large sheet of paper, and carry out your own computations with a portable calculator? (Rough guide: okay if say 50 subjects and 20 variables.)
2. What statistical tests are you going to use? (You'd better learn about them, and the assumptions that each one makes about the data, as soon as possible.)
3. Do you need statistical advice? Unless you are wholly exceptional, the answer to this question is 'YES'. If you have access to a medical statistician, rough out what you intend to do and the tests you intend to use and ask for his or her comments. Don't ask for help after the fieldwork is complete. ("If I was going to Chipping Sodbury, I wouldn't have started from here".)

Title:

Psychiatric screening tests and the Medical Interview.

Aim:

What is the relationship between scores on a psychiatric screening test and cues which might indicate psychological distress in a subsequent medical interview?

It is known that a substantial proportion of patients in primary care settings with high scores do not complain about psychological symptoms: the study will discover to what extent such patients give non-verbal and vocal cues suggesting illness, and which particular cues are strongly related to emotional distress.

Method:

The study will use existing videotapes of encounters between GP vocational trainees and patients who have previously completed the GHQ-28 which exist in the Department. A colleague will select interviews in such a way that each score band on the GHQ is represented equally, and these interviews will be rated by the investigator without knowledge of the GHQ scores. Each interview will be rated twice: first without sound in order to rate non-verbal cues; then with sound in order to rate vocal and verbal cues relating to psychological distress. Six patients will be rated in each of the eight following score-bands:
0/ 1-4 (threshold!)/ 5-8/ 9-12/ 13-16/ 17-20/ 21-24/ 25-28

A pilot study using interviews which have not been selected for the main study will familiarize the investigator with the rating procedures, and will be followed by a small inter-rater reliability study with a worker who has already used the scales on other projects.

Measures:

The investigator will use existing scales in the Department for rating non-verbal cues and vocal cues relating to psychological distress. Ratings will be made of the first 5 minutes of each encounter at the end of each minute, using 13 non-verbal cues, and four types of verbal cue. Each cue is rated on a 3-point scale.

Ethical aspects:

There are no ethical problems: all patients have given informed consent for the recordings to be made and used for teaching and research purposes.

Treatment of results:

These will be presented graphically to investigate the relationship between score level and each cue. Relationships between score level and cues will be tested using analysis of variance. With only 48 subjects, the data will be processed by hand.

Fig. 20.1. An example of a research protocol

Title and aim

You can now make last-minute adjustments to your title, and to your all-important 'aim'. An example of a research protocol is shown in Figure 20.1.

Take your research protocol to your supervisor, and expect to have to make modifications to it in the light of criticisms: don't expect to have got it right first time!

OBTAINING MONEY

Most small projects can be achieved by using office supplies that are available in most departments of psychiatry. If your project needs equipment that costs money, or will involve you in extra travel expenses, ask your supervisor if any funds exist that might give you assistance.

THE PROJECT LOG

You start this as soon as your protocol has been agreed to by a more experienced person – usually your supervisor. Like the notebook which preceded it, it must be small enough to be carried about with you. You still have a section for jotting down references to papers relevant to your project, but most of it is in diary form.

The time budget

This vital, but somewhat depressing page, should be right at the front. Put today's date on the top line, and the date when the project must be finished and submitted on the bottom. (In the example which follows, we will assume that you are preparing a Master's dissertation.)

You start from the bottom and work up:

- You must allow six weeks for your supervisor to read the final manuscript, for you to make alterations, and for the binder to bind the dissertation.

- Writing the final manuscript, even if you make a start a year before submission date, should have three clear months allowed for it.
- The time allowed for calculations and data analyses depend very much upon the complexity of your project: an average would be three months, however!
- The Main study: try to decide how long this will take, and then allow a generous time margin for illness, holidays, refusals, poor collaboration from colleagues, and things going wrong generally.
- The Pilot study: do you need one? (see below)
- Training period: you almost certainly aren't ready to start tomorrow – allow time for instruments to be obtained, and for you to familiarize yourself with them. You may need special training in order to administer a research interview – allow time for this.
- Gaining ethical approval: fortunately you can be training yourself while you wait for this.

Having done this, you may find yourself with a few months to spare. Congratulations – but you'll probably need it. However, it is more likely that you'll find that you have a negative amount of time. In this case you revise your budget, trimming off a month here and there, and remembering that there is no time to be lost from now on.

In the remainder of the project log you write notes with appropriate dates: when you come to write up your 'method' and 'results' it is in your project log that you find the dates when the main study started and stopped, or the serial number of a patient who illustrated some particular point. You will record full details of refusals to co-operate, of people not included for various reasons who should have been, and if appropriate details of total numbers of patients from which a sample was drawn on a particular day.

THE PILOT STUDY

This tests the acceptability and practicality of your proposed procedure for both patients and any other staff who may be involved. It familiarizes others with your procedures, and allows you to adjust both methods and procedures in the light of experience in the field. You can also use a pilot study to determine the variances in your main measures in order to decide how large a group of subjects you will need.

The main study is deemed to have begun only when you decide to make no further alterations in the procedures and measures that are to be used.

Make sure that you are recording data in a way that will enable you to score any research interviews more easily at the end of the study. If you decide to use a standardized research interview or to administer a questionnaire, make sure that you use the original forms: it is invalid to construct your own 'shorthand' set of ratings, ignoring the format of the instrument from which the ratings were derived.

Some research projects involve you in recording the patients' replies to open questions. If there are only a small number of possible replies to a particular question, you will of course 'pre-code' the replies, and just mark the appropriate response on your form. Most people think of that. However, if you cannot anticipate all possible replies, although you can be fairly sure of some of them, remember that you can 'partially pre-code' a question. Here you are still free to write down in longhand anything that your patients say that doesn't fit into the pre-coded responses, but you will have to go through all such responses at the end of the study and decide what natural groups the replies fall into. This is called 'post-coding'. Try to reduce the amount of this, as you will find that it is very time-consuming.

THE MAIN STUDY

On the day you start this the time for original thought is over: most projects merely involve humdrum work from now on. You should also start the writing up of the project at about this time. Write the *Method* first: you can't change anything from now on, and there will be no better time to write it. Go straight on to the *Literature Review*, and aim to finish this during the main study.

If time is running short, and you have a large data set, remember that it can be very useful to start data analyses before data collection is completed. This gives you an opportunity to decide on the exact tests you are going to carry out, and perhaps to get the data you have so far onto a computer. Once you have a program running smoothly, it is a very simple matter to add the last few cases and to carry out the final data run.

DATA PROCESSING

Many small projects will be carried out on your desk with the aid of a calculator. It is very useful indeed to plot all your data yourself, by hand, on a large sheet of paper. You may see things that would never have struck you if your data had been put straight into a computer by someone else.

Don't rush to carry out statistical tests. Gloat over your data a bit; plot it on squared paper, draw it in histograms, try various cross-tabulations.

Don't make a fool of yourself by carrying out statistical tests on data that are obviously null. If your data fall just short of statistical significance, and there is still time, consider adding a few cases to your main study. (It may well make no difference!) If your data show a large difference but your (double-checked!) statistical test shows it not to be significant, consult someone more experienced. It may well be that you have made an error in your calculation, or they may be able to suggest an alternative statistical treatment for your data.

Large data sets

Ideally, you should aim to learn to use a computer terminal yourself, so that you can do what you like with your own data. If others are responsible for coding and entering your data, it is vital that once the data is entered it is 'verified' by someone else: this means that it is entered again, so that any mistakes can be rectified. (It is unusual for the same mistake to be made by two different people.)

Once the data is safely inside the computer it is a good plan to ask for a 'Data Listing', which is merely a print-out showing you your raw data as they have been fed into the computer. You should ask for the 'frequencies' of all your variables.

Before you become engrossed in your cross-tabulations, spend a little time checking the quality of your data. Are the right totals shown in the main cells? If you happen to know what one of the variables should be, does the computer agree with you? You will often find that it does not. This almost certainly means that there have been mistakes either in coding the data, or in entering it into the computer. The time-consuming but vital business of *cleaning the data* now begins: you find the offending variable on your data listing, place a long straight-edge along it, and scan for impossible values or missing values. If you don't find any, the tedium of checking each patient has to be undertaken. Cleaning a large data set may take several weeks, but you are wasting your time with dirty data.

WRITING UP YOUR PROJECT

Your final manuscript will be in the following order: title page; contents; abstract; acknowledgments; and then the following chapters: Introduction; Literature Review; Method; Results; Discussion. These are written in the following order:

Method

Don't bother to give full descriptions of tests that have already been published, unless they are little known tests dug out of obscure journals. In the latter case, it is wise not only to describe them, but to reproduce them in an Appendix. Any measuring instrument designed specially for the study must be described in detail, giving reasons for any features that may not be self-evident. Details of the number of patients in each group, and how many refusals you encountered, are 'results', not 'method'.

The Literature Review

When you feel ready to start this draw a diagram of the review – show what subheadings you intend to use, jot down the main arguments that will be developed in each section. Then show it to your supervisor. Most beginners cram far too much into their literature reviews, and include turgid accounts of things that need not be described in great detail. Your supervisor may save you a lot of trouble at this supervision. Remember that a literature review should build up to a climax, so that the reader is left eagerly anticipating the study they are about to read: one tries to suggest that the subject of the dissertation is one that addresses an important, and unresolved, matter.

Results

This starts with full details of the field work: when it started and stopped, where it was carried out, how the sample studied may have differed from the larger population from which it was drawn. Remember to give full details about refusals, and to show if you had to depart from your original intentions.

Don't try to say things in words that are better shown in numbers, but write an accompanying text which reads well by itself. Don't show unnecessary tables, which cannot possibly advance the argument put forward by your research. DON'T, on any account, give results to eight decimal places simply because the computer did, and don't fall into the pernicious practice of giving significance levels without showing what values you found in the data. The section on 'results' ends with a clear summary reminding the reader what has been shown. Be careful not to include any evaluations or discussion of your results at this stage.

Discussion

Your literature review ended with a summary of the state of knowledge of your particular topic; your results ended with a succinct statement of your findings. In the discussion, you merely discuss the latter in the light of the former. Be critical about any positive findings, and refute them yourself if you can – far better you than someone else! But there is no need to be over-critical.

Introduction

The most difficult thing to write of all, undoubtedly best left until the end, when you know what you have shown. It describes the problem which is to be the subject of the dissertation in rather general terms, without entering into a review of the literature, or anticipating the actual results of the enquiry. You won't get it right first time.

Abstract

This is an anti-climax after the ordeal of the introduction, but logically it is best left until the end (200 words maximum!).

PREPARING FOR PUBLICATION

Oddly enough, this is much easier after you have written your dissertation, since one can be clearer about what can be left out. Decide on your journal of first choice, and write in its house-style and no longer than an average article in that journal.

I am grateful to Dr Graeme McGrath for making valuable comments on an earlier draft of this chapter.

Further reading

Sainsbury P and Kreitman N (1975) *Methods of Psychiatric Research, 2nd edition.* London: Oxford University Press

— 21

A North American Perspective

Graham Glancy

The purpose of this chapter is to discuss a number of issues which are important and topical in North American psychiatric training. Some of these topics such as psychiatric morbidity in trainees are equally relevant to British psychiatry but are not covered in the preceding chapters.

The majority of the chapters in this book are equally applicable on both sides of the Atlantic. However, areas where there are significant differences include: the content of psychiatric rotations, diagnostic classification, examinations and some of the legal aspects of practice.

PSYCHIATRIC ROTATIONS

One essential difference between training on the two sides of the Atlantic is the truncation of the training period on the North American continent. The standard length of a "residency programme" is four years, although this may be even shorter if the trainee has experience in a related field, for instance a year in general practice or a related medical speciality or if he has a degree in a field such as sociology, neuropharmacology or psychology. In these cases, it may only be necessary to spend three years as a resident. The vital point is that after this period you are entitled to practise as a fully qualified psychiatrist or consultant once you have passed the specialists' examination. However, this is too short a period and the trainee should still take advantage of at least four years of training before taking on the responsibilities of a fully trained psychiatrist.

Fellowship programmes offer a chance to increase the training period and are especially, but not exclusively, useful for the person who wants to follow a career in a subspeciality. They are also particularly appropriate for an academic career. A fellowship programme should follow a generic training where at least a minimum core of necessary knowledge and skills have been learned and demonstrated. These programmes are usually offered in a university setting. They offer an invaluable opportunity to concentrate on the subspeciality and may also provide the opportunity to participate in a research project in this area. "Diplomate" examinations may be available as the natural culmination of this year, and they may give the trainee some recognition of his endeavour.

In some ways, a fellowship is analogous to the SR position in the UK. As well as providing valuable training there are other distinctive advantages to these programmes. Firstly, you can discover whether you really enjoy the speciality at a stage where it is easier to leave if you find that full-time involvement in this speciality is after all not what you want. Secondly, you are in an ideal position to make contacts regarding future appointments and to hear about and compare facilities at various places.

When choosing a psychiatric rotation, it is necessary to tread carefully through the bewildering quagmire of considerations. It is essential to be aware of the requirements laid down by the relevant governing body at state or provincial levels as well as at federal levels. In Canada, many rotations are having to accommodate recent Royal College amendments involving chronic care placements, consultation–liaison posts and general hospital experience. As well as satisfying the requirements of the appropriate legislative body, you have to maximize the learning opportunities available and choose a rotation which will best equip you for the type of position you eventually envisage yourself settling in. A reasonable balance between the psychodynamic and organic orientations should be achieved by choosing appropriate placements. This point raises some controversy. A recent study of all psychiatrists in the state of Washington found that 40 per cent of psychiatrists described their practice as "analytic", 27 per cent as "dynamic", 14 per cent as "biological", 8 per cent as "cognitive" and 3 per cent as "existential". In their conclusions, the authors noted that "very little in-patient work was done", and questioned the requirements of the American Psychiatric Association that "one year whole" is spent on an in-patient unit. A recent meeting of the staff of one facility debated this very issue in response to pressure by some trainees who felt that they would benefit from a training programme which emphasized psychodynamic out-patient experience designed to prepare them for private practice. The staff at this meeting unanimously decided that the current emphasis on multi-theoretical and multi-treatment approaches should continue to provide the "core" of the training experience.

Discussions with the postgraduate co-ordinator (tutor), fellow residents who are perhaps further on in training, as well as qualified psychiatrists, especially those in the field where you have a special interest, are very useful in helping choose placements in the context of the relevant legislation. Be careful not to put all your eggs in one basket, for instance by doing the maximum possible out-patient and psychotherapeutic posts, only to find that after four years of training you have decided that private practice or a wholly psychotherapeutic practice is not suitable for you.

SUPERVISION

Psychotherapy supervision is an essential part of any psychiatric training. As well as supervision of a short-term patient, long-term supervision is also essential. As this requires longer than the supervision provided by a supervisor in a six-month placement, arrangements should be made to "take with you" one or more patients whilst ensuring continuity of supervision of the work with these patients. This supervision is necessary for learning the fundamentals of psychodynamic theory as well as the practice of therapy whilst experiencing the trials and tribulations of treating a long-term patient. This can be a most rewarding and enriching experience.

Supervision may touch on some of the trainee's own neurotic conflicts, and he must be able to discuss these with his supervisor. One of the most difficult realizations and transitions from physician to trainee psychiatrist is the fact that we may all have unresolved neurotic conflicts and, even more startling, it is not always necessary to deny these. In fact, in some circumstances, these may best be dealt with in personal therapy. Psychotherapy supervision, however, should be clearly differentiated from personal therapy, and if the supervisor–trainee dyad sometimes treads the fine line between treatment and supervision, it should definitely not cross this line. If a trainee feels that he needs personal therapy, he should make this decision for himself and make the necessary arrangements, perhaps in consultation with psychotherapy supervisor and postgraduate co-ordinator. In North America psychotherapy does not carry the stigma that it does in Britain, and in fact may be viewed as a sign that the trainee is able to recognize affect and conflict within himself without denial. By personally experiencing the beneficial effects of therapy, he may find that this helps him reaffirm his confidence in psychiatry. This is further discussed below.

Groups

Various types of groups are available for trainees in various settings. In Toronto an annual T-group is run for all trainees. The T-group traditionally focuses on identity issues, resolution of conflict and treatment of interpersonal problems. In the training setting, this may not be appropriate and may actually contribute to morbidity. Salvendy states that if the goals of the group are clearly defined then the unwanted effects can be countered. Amongst the goals should be the production of an awareness of group psychodynamic principles at the same time steering away from treatment issues. Experienced group leaders are necessary to facilitate these principles. These groups may be regular or periodic, each of which has both advantages and disadvantages.

Another type of group is the so-called "study group". This group meets regularly and focuses on clearly defined educational topics. It can be formal or informal. One format involves the discussion of old examination questions on a weekly basis. Often the questions are so obscure that it requires the resources of a group to decide on an answer. This is a useful experience and can make the necessary but arduous task of ploughing through old examinations quite enjoyable.

The apprenticeship model

The apprenticeship model of supervision is still invaluable and a *sine qua non* of clinical training. Supervision may focus on the patient (cf Caplan's client-orientated consultation) or upon the trainee (consultant orientated consultation) but is usually a combination of both within a supervisory alliance. Supervision is both formal and informal and constitutes such elements as advice, validation, modelling and support. It is helpful to set aside a formal time of one to two hours on a weekly basis so that both the trainee and supervisor can focus on specific issues in supervision. One of the most difficult problems a trainee has to face is how to deal with a jaded, incompetent or excessively busy supervisor. It is here that the postgraduate co-ordinator (tutor) can be of help in liaising with the supervisor so as to help remedy the situation. Of course, the trainee also has a role in actively seeking supervision and being available to the supervisor. Many trainees go through a period analogous to adolescent rebellion when they resent supervision and avoid their supervisors. This phase should be recognized by both supervisor and trainee and dealt with appropriately as a healthy developmental process.

PSYCHIATRIC ILLNESS IN TRAINEES

Estimates of psychiatric morbidity in trainees range from four to 25 per cent. Kelly surveyed a group of programme directors and found that four per cent of trainees committed or attempted suicide or had disabilities "of sufficient intensity to require special treatment or hospitalization". A recent self-report questionnaire at the University of Toronto suggested that 25 per cent of trainees were moderately to severely depressed. This figure, in accord with others, showed that the highest incidence of depression was amongst first-year trainees and amongst females. This is not, as many may erroneously surmise, solely a North American phenomenon. In one British study Waring found that 22 per cent of psychiatric trainees had a score on the GHQ in the range of highly probable non-psychotic emotional illness. Other studies have suggested that high-risk factors may include:

- Being in the first year.
- Age greater than 30.
- Marital status – single or divorced.
- Being female.
- Graduation from a foreign medical school.
- Transfers from another programme.
- Race or ethnic group.

Many authors suggest that psychiatric training is a particular type of emotional stressor. Some use the term "role-shock" to describe the conflict that the trainee experiences when "giving up the stethoscope". In addition to this, there is a variety of other stresses, some of which are peculiar to psychiatric training and some of which are general to medical training, the practice of medicine or to other postgraduate experience. Much of the stress may be alleviated later in the residency so that an initial reaction should not be taken as evidence of emotional disturbance severe enough to warrant exclusion from further training. The trainee should, therefore, be aware of these stresses and anxieties and recognize them as a common and perhaps even essential aspect of training. If he is satisfactorily able to work through them, then this may represent evidence of the personal growth and self-understanding necessary for development as a psychiatrist.

Intervention may be at the level of increasing support, supervision and attention to the morale and cohesion amongst the trainee peer group. Personal therapy, as discussed above, may also be an option. Between 50 and 70 per cent of trainees in North America will enter psychotherapy of some kind during their training period. Clearly, the more disturbed the trainee, the more compelling the case for therapy. Personal therapy is considered essential by some psychiatrists. Others consider it desirable but it is rarely looked upon as a sign of weakness or a sign that the trainee is inappropriate for continuation in the scheme.

CLASSIFICATION

The American Psychiatric Association has adopted DSM-III as its official diagnostic classification. In Canada, both DSM-III and ICD-9 are equally acceptable and it is necessary to be conversant with both. Increasingly, however, DSM-III is becoming more generally used, particularly where research criteria or statistical use of the diagnoses is intended. DSM-III explains and justifies itself in its own introduction and appendices and amplification is available in any recently published North American textbook. DSM-III uses operational rather than purely descriptive criteria for diagnosis. It also uses a multi-axial system which can be useful, although axes III and IV are primarily intended for research.

When used sensibly, it is a useful tool. Like any tool, it depends upon the expertise of the operator. Amongst its pitfalls, the trainee should be aware that some entities are new and have yet to be extensively validated. Schizotypal personality disorder is an example of this. Another potential pitfall is the use of a check list or cook book approach to "prove" a diagnosis without careful clinical assessment.

Laymen, such as lawyers, are particularly at risk here and the psychiatric trainee should not follow their example. This classification is not intended to obviate careful clinical examination and diagnostic acumen. Another problem is that the lack of an aetiological approach may lead to a failure to question why the patient presents in a particular manner. This question is an essential part of the formulation.

Trainees should acquaint themselves with both diagnostic systems. They should also be aware of the antecedents to each system and their respective historical development.

Having done that, be prepared for DSM-IIIR, which will be produced in early 1987. Be prepared for such diagnoses as "self-defeating personality disorder", "paraphilic cohesive disorder" and "pre-menstrual dysphoric disorder".

RESEARCH

Goldberg's quotation, prefacing his chapter (p.252), is crisp and apposite. However, how is a trainee to develop the skills and knowledge necessary to embark upon research on his own? When is there time to fit this into the busy schedule of lectures, seminars and service commitments, including on call? The answer lies in choosing the rotation which provides an integrated approach to research training within a general clinical programme. The trainee should in addition avail himself of every opportunity to learn about research. Journal clubs, research presentations and conferences, as well as a regular perusal of current literature, all give essential exposure to research and go hand-in-hand with a research training programme. According to McGuire and Fairbanks, this programme should emphasize early exposure to research faculty in a clinical setting, an early focus on research, special research seminars and options for participation in a research project. Personal participation from an early stage is most important, and the trainee should consider research as an important part of his training. He should, therefore, be prepared to allot himself suitable time for research just as he would for clinical duties or administration. There is always an excuse *not* to do research. It is also necessary to speak up for reasonable clerical and material support. With a good research training, the trainee should develop a competency to access research data in a critical manner, if only so as to be able to apply this data to clinical practice and current ideas.

AUDIT

Although the concept of medical audit is by no means new on either side of the Atlantic, it is well instituted in North America. Many hospitals have audit committees which may comprise strictly medical staff or the members of the multi-disciplinary team. A multi-disciplinary team audit committee may not only audit suicidal and violent incidents, but also have a mandate to audit the quality of recording and practice in general. For instance, it may carry out retrospective or "spot" audits on "the pre-lithium work-up" and also the "pre-ECT work-up" as well as checking the frequency that a particular form, such as that regarding financial competence, is correctly filled out. This committee reports directly to the medical advisory committee, which makes appropriate recommendations. There is no doubt that this is a useful procedure and helps to maintain high standards.

Any trainee who has the opportunity to join this committee should take the opportunity, as it is a valuable educational experience.

LEGAL ISSUES

The United States is a relatively new country which is based on a legislated constitution. This is one of the reasons that its legislation has developed by a process of constant recourse to the judiciary for clarification and modification. Legal issues, therefore, seem more in the forefront of one's mind when practising in North America. Apart from the well-known issue of "malpractice", as it is known, the issues of informed consent and confidentiality are worthy of discussion. Malpractice needs no further comment, except to say, as in any jurisdiction, that good clinical care, appropriate recording, the taking of reasonable precautions, and according to one's level of responsibility, appropriate consultation makes the doctor immune from prosecution.

"Informed consent" is a multi-faceted doctrine which has two goals: (1) to promote individual autonomy, and (2) to encourage rational decision-making.

According to Lidz and colleagues there are five basic issues:

- Information
- Understanding
- Competency
- Voluntariness
- Decision-making

The application of this doctrine to psychiatry raises a number of difficulties which are discussed in Lidz's work. Each issue listed has its own problems but, in psychiatry, the issues of understanding, competency, voluntariness and decision-making may all be profoundly affected by mental illness. At the forefront of the controversy is consent to ECT.

Recent Canadian and American decisions have rejected the "reasonable medical standard" when deciding on the amount of information to disclose. Instead the standard is the amount of information that a reasonable person in that patient's shoes would have wanted in order to be able to make an informed decision.

The British position is somewhat different. In a recent case the House of Lords held that the amount of information a doctor gives should be decided by the doctor, as long as his decision is not in conflict with accepted and responsible medical practice.

If the trainee in North America does not comply with the

accepted doctrine, then he makes himself vulnerable to censure. A similar civil libertarian approach applies to research consent and even questionnaires are now considered to be in some respects invasive. Recourse and advice from the appropriate ethics review committee are mandatory before undertaking any research project.

The trainee should also be aware of the standards of confidentiality in the jurisdiction where he will be training. In Ontario, for instance, one cannot provide any information about a patient to another professional or a relative without signed consent of the patient on the appropriate form of the Mental Health Act. In the case of an incompetent patient, the consent of a next-of-kin is legal. Although this can be cumbersome, it does serve to safeguard the patient's rights and confidentiality. This confidentiality can only be broken in particular circumstances, such as a life-and-death emergency, for example when a comatose patient is brought into the Emergency Room. Another situation where confidentiality can be broken is when child abuse is suspected. In Ontario, it is legislated that it is *mandatory* for any physician to notify the local services if such abuse is suspected. Another circumstance where confidentiality must be broken arises out of the case of *Tarasoff v Regents of the University of California.* In this case, Poddar, a psychotherapy out-patient at the University of California, told his psychotherapist of his fantasy of killing Tatiana Tarasoff. The psychologist was concerned and informed the campus police who questioned Poddar and warned him to stay away from the young lady. However, he went and killed her. Her family sued the university including the police and therapists. The court held that the psychologist has a duty to warn the intended victims. Over the last 12 years, this ruling has been debated by the courts, culminating in the introduction of Bill 1133 of the California Assembly which clarifies the issue, stating "where the patient has communicated to the psychotherapist, a serious threat of violence against a reasonably identifiable victim . . . that duty may be discharged by making . . . reasonable efforts to communicate the threat to the victim and to a law enforcement agency".

This case has been interpreted differently by courts in different states and it is a priority to know the position in the jurisdiction where you are practising. You should not be afraid to seek consultation or supervision in cases where doubt exists.

LICENSING AND EXAMINATIONS

Both Canada and the United States are large countries whose bureaucracy is compounded by the fact that both provinces (or states) and the Federal Legislature must have their say. Each jurisdiction, therefore, has its own licensing requirement which will have to be satisfied in conjunction with the federal requirements. Anybody considering a post in North America should contact the postgraduate co-ordinator as well as the state and federal licensing bodies about these requirements. All three contacts are necessary since it is possible to be misled by one or the other. Full knowledge of these requirements prior to accepting any post can sometimes be followed by negotiations. Trainees from abroad may be able to do without one or other requirement, particularly if they are applying for a government or state position or if the employers particularly want them for the job. The trainee should, however, be prepared to take the minimal licensure requirements such as Flex, VQE, ECFMG, or LMCC if he wants later to take a permanent post in North America. If he is only intending to spend a part of his training period in North America, he may be able to escape without these hurdles. Specialists' examinations will also be necessary for the trainee considering taking a consultant position in North America.

However, these examinations are not identical to the MRCPsych. The style and format of the exam and any peculiarities that it might have should be carefully studied.

The trainee should also practise by using previous years' papers and "mock orals" in order to adapt to different styles and techniques of interviewing and formulating.

Further reading

Beck JC (1985) *The Potentially Violent Patient and the Tarasoff Decision in Psychiatric Practice.* Washington, DC: American Psychiatric Press

Campbell HD (1982) Prevalence and ramifications of psychopathology in psychiatric residents: an overview. *American Journal of Psychiatry 139:* 1405–1411

Kelly WA (1973) Suicide and psychiatric education. *American Journal of Psychiatry 130:* 463–468

Lidz CW, Meisel E, Zerubarrel E, Carter M, Sestak RM and Roth LH (1984) *Informed Consent: A Study of Decision-making in Psychiatry.* New York: Guildford

Salvendy JT and Steward MF (1983) Training groups in residents. *Journal of Psychiatric Education 7:* 287–295

Schuster DB, Sandt JJ and Tholer OF (1972) *Clinical Supervision of the Psychiatric Resident.* New York: Brunner: Mozzel

Webb LJ, DiClemente CC, Johnstone EE, Sanders JL and Perley RA, eds (1981) *DSM-III Training Guide: For use with APA Diagnostic and Statistical Manual of Mental Disorders, 3rd edition.* New York: Brunner: Mozzel

A Glossary of Some Important Terms in Psychiatry

Affect (syn. mood) – a patient's emotional state; it has a subjective component which takes the form of feelings which each person can recognize in himself (e.g. unhappiness) and an objective component which is the outward manifestations of the feelings (e.g. sad facial expression; dejected posture).
Lability of affect – a heightened tendency for affect to fluctuate or for one mood to change rapidly to another.
Inappropriate (syn. incongruous) affect – emotion not in keeping with the circumstances or what is expected.
Blunting of affect – an apparent restriction or lack of normal emotional responsiveness, as judged by expressionless face and voice, indifference to distressing topics and apathy.
Agitation – increased motor activity with a background of marked anxiety, e.g. fidgeting, restlessness, constantly shifting posture, wringing hands, pacing up and down.
Ambivalence – vacillation between complying and refusing when asked to do something; also refers to vacillation of motivation.
Anxiety – (see also 'Tension') the affect of fear, apprehension or a sense of danger; consciousness may be narrowed so that thinking is restricted to the object of anxiety; symptoms and signs of autonomic nervous system overactivity may be present: blushing, butterflies, choking, diarrhoea, difficulty getting breath, dizziness, dry mouth, giddiness, palpitations, sweating, trembling, weakness at the knees.
Anxious foreboding – the unjustified feeling that something terrible is going to happen, e.g. disaster, illness, ruination, but patient perhaps not sure what.
Free-floating anxiety – the existence or persistence of anxious mood, with or without autonomic activity, in the absence of provoking or persisting thoughts or circumstances.
Phobic anxiety – anxiety, tension or panic which occurs in certain situations irrationally, e.g. meeting other people (social phobia), leaving the security of one's own home and mixing in crowds (agoraphobia), being confined in places such as lifts or tube trains (claustrophobia) or particular animals such as spiders, snakes and cats and particular situations such as air travel (the specific phobias); the patient typically avoids the situations that provoke anxiety ('phobic avoidance').
Approximate answers – responses to questions which consistently just miss being correct and imply a knowledge of the correct answer.

Autistic thinking – fantasizing.
Automatic obedience – undue compliance with instructions, e.g. the patient's movements can be guided by the pressure of one finger.
Automatism – a simple or complex motor act, often inappropriate to the situation, carried out while unaware of the environment, e.g. undressing in supermarket after epileptic seizure.
Belle indifference – the presentation of distressing disabilities with no obvious accompanying emotional disturbance.
Catastrophic reaction – an explosive expression of affect which occurs when a patient attempts a task beyond his capabilities.
Catatonic phenomena – a collective term for a variety of motor behaviours including automatic obedience, echophenomena, ambivalence, negativism, posturing and waxy flexibility.
Circumstantiality – long-winded, pedantic speech with many unnecessary details but the goal remains in sight and is eventually reached.
Clouding of consciousness – a diminution of level of consciousness as evidenced by a diffuse impairment of cognitive functions, a reduced and fluctuating awareness of the environment, diminished grasp, drowsiness and an increased threshold for incoming stimuli; if hallucinations and psychomotor agitation are also present the state may be called 'delirium'.
Compulsive acts – actions which have to be carried out a number of times in spite of attempts to resist the desire and in the knowledge that the act may be absurd; failure to carry out the act results in anxiety.
Concretization – the interpretation of abstract ideas in a literal manner.
Confabulation – changing, loosely held falsified memories which fill gaps of memory in an organically-determined amnesia. The patient has no insight into his amnesia.
Conflict – the presence of two or more incompatible aims, particularly repressed childhood wishes in opposition to the need to function as an adult in society.
Delirium – see 'Clouding of consciousness'.
Delusion – false belief held with total conviction and inappropriate to the patient's intelligence, social background and subcultural beliefs.
Delusional mood – the feeling that something in the environment has changed in a strange, odd or puzzling way, which cannot be described and is specially significant for the patient.
Delusional perception – the attribution of an unexplained, new and personal meaning to a normal perception.
Autochthonous delusion – a fully-formed delusion which suddenly appears in the patient's mind.
Primary (syn. true) delusion – a delusion which is not psychologically understandable, is held with extraordinary conviction and is impervious to counter argument.

Secondary delusion – a delusion which can be understood as deriving from an existing disturbance of affect, perception or personality.

Depersonalization – a feeling of being unreal, acting a part rather than being spontaneous and natural, being a sham, a shadow of a real person or detached from one's experiences.

Depression – the affect of sadness, misery, dejection or grief.

Derealization – an experience of the surroundings as being unreal or like a stage with actors, the surroundings may seem colourless, artificial or dead.

Echophenomena – the automatic imitation of movements (echopraxia) or speech (echolalia).

Ecstasy – a feeling of rapture and extreme joy which may be accompanied by the feeling that the riddles of life or problems of mankind have been solved (see 'Elation' and 'Euphoria').

Elation – states of well-being, optimism, cheerfulness, which are normal.

Euphoria – responses to achievements and good news but morbid when they are out of keeping with the situation.

Flight of ideas – a disorder, manifested in speech, in which the patient wanders from one theme to another on the basis of a variety of verbal associations (assonance, punning, rhyme/slang associations) or according to distracting stimuli; the speech lacks direction; the tempo is usually, but not invariably, increased.

Free association – a technique developed by Freud which encourages the patient to state freely whatever comes to mind however fragmentary and seemingly illogical. Through the associations revealed it is possible to detect repressed areas of conflict.

Fugue – a sudden disturbance of behaviour characterized by a tendency to wander; associated with altered or impaired consciousness and subsequent partial or total amnesia.

Hallucination – a false perception lacking an adequate basis in external stimuli.

Hopelessness – a negative view of the future experienced as a feeling that there is no point going on; when present in mild degree the patient may behave as if hope remains, but when present in severe degree the patient may neglect himself and his affairs.

Hypochondriasis – an abnormal preoccupation with ill-health which is real, imagined or anticipated.

Ideas of reference – the idea that events (e.g. the words or actions of other people) refer especially to the patient when, in reality, they have no such significance.

Illusion – a false perception based on the misinterpretation of a real stimulus.

Interpretation – intervention by the therapist directed to making unconscious material conscious.

Irritability – the experience of poor control over temper leading to verbal or physical expressions of anger.
Made experiences – emotions, drives or volition experienced as being made by an outside impulse, i.e. made feelings, made impulses, made acts.
Mannerisms – idiosyncratic and repeated variations in goal-directed movements which are so pronounced that they may appear odd or stilted, e.g. unusual hand movements when shaking hands, saluting three times before entering a room.
Mental mechanisms – assumed modes of mental functioning which would account for clinical observations particularly such phenomena as repression (qv).
Negativism – a purposeless refusal to obey instructions or the performance of the exact opposite of what is asked.
Neologism – a new word specially constructed by the patient and often forming part of a private language.
Obsession – an unpleasant thought, causing great anxiety, which cannot be driven from consciousness, which repeatedly intrudes into the mind in spite of attempts to resist it and which is recognized as senseless but recognized as the patient's own thought.
Over-valued idea – a thought, or collection of thoughts, which are given precedence over others, dominate the conscious life, are associated with much affect, usually negative and are comprehensible in the light of past experiences and the personality of the subject.
Panic attack – a discrete episode of intense fear and anxiety, with autonomic accompaniments, which the patients seeks to terminate by some drastic but appropriate avoiding action, e.g. rushing outside for air, rushing to a neighbour.
Passivity experience – the false belief that the patient is the passive and unwilling recipient of the control by and influence of an alien force which penetrates the subject's mind or body.
Perplexity – the association of a puzzled expression with a state of bewilderment and an inability to understand what is happening.
Perseveration – the persistence of a motor, verbal or ideational response after it has ceased to be appropriate.
Phobia – a fear which is out of proportion to the situation or object, cannot be explained or reasoned away, is beyond voluntary control and leads to avoidance of the feared situation or object (see 'Anxiety, phobic').
Posturing – the exhibition of abnormal posture.
Manneristic posture – an odd, stilted posture which is an exaggeration of a normal one and not rigidly preserved.
Stereotyped posture – an abnormal and non-adaptive posture which is rigidly maintained and often uncomfortable.
Preservation of posture – the maintenance for long periods of postures which have arisen fortuitously or been imposed by the examiner.

Pressure of speech – speech that is excessive in speed or quantity or both.

Prolixity – a mild form of pressure of speech.

Pseudo-hallucination – a form of abnormal perception characterized by the experience of a false precept in inner subjective space and lacking the vividness, depth and constancy of a true hallucination; it may have an 'as if' quality.

Repression – the active removal from consciousness of painful thoughts and feelings.

Resistance – forces within the patient which oppose the treatment process. More specifically in psychodynamic therapy, forces which lead to distortions and disguise of unconscious impulses and wishes.

Retardation – the morbid slowing of thought processes and movements.

Speeding of thoughts – the experience of thoughts entering the mind and proceeding at increased speed; in extreme degree the thoughts are experienced as crowding in.

Stereotyped behaviour – utterances or movements which are monotonously repeated, non-goal directed, executed in a uniform way and do not seem to have any special significance for the patient, e.g. rocking to and fro on chair, rubbing head round and round with hand, grimacing.

Stupor (akinetic mutism) – a state of almost complete absence of movement and speech with preservation of consciousness inferred from ocular fixation.

Tension

Muscular tension – an unpleasant and uncomfortable increase in muscle tension which may be localized or widespread.

Nervous tension – the feeling of being on edge, mentally tense or under a nervous strain.

Thought block – the sudden cessation of a train of thought, unrelated to increased arousal or anxiety and resulting in a complete but brief absence of thoughts.

Thought broadcasting – the delusion that the subject's private thoughts are being made known to and shared with others.

Thought echo – the experience of thoughts being repeated or echoed with very little interval between the original and the echo.

Thought insertion – the subject experiences the intrusion into his mind of thoughts which are definitely not his own and which may be attributed to some alien person or power.

Thought withdrawal – the subject exhibits the delusion that his thoughts are being removed from his head so that he has no thoughts, the removal may be attributed to an alien person or power.

Torpor – a state or pathological awareness; drowsiness with a tendency to fall into a dreamless sleep.

Transference – feelings which had their origins in earlier life repeated in the relationship with the therapist. This process, initially unconscious, is brought into awareness during the treatment.

Twilight state – conscious awareness is narrowed down to a few ideas and attitudes which dominate the patient's mind.

Unconscious – in psychoanalytic theory seen as the original mode of mental functioning (using primary process thinking, displacement, and condensation and with a disregard for chronology). Also the repository for thoughts and feelings removed from consciousness by repression.

Waxy flexibility – a feeling of plastic resistance, like bending a soft wax rod, when the examiner moves the patient's body; the posture may be preserved when the passive movement stops.

Appendix

AN INDEX TO SOME ICD–9 DISORDERS*

Affective psychoses	
alcoholic mania NOS	291.9
manic depressive psychosis	296.0–296.9
mixed affective state	296.4
mixed paranoid and affective organic psychosis	294.8
reactive depressive psychosis	298.0
reactive excitative/manic psychosis	298.1
schizoaffective psychosis	295.7
Alcohol-related disorders	
dementia	291.2
dependence syndrome	303
intoxication	305.0
Korsakoff's syndrome	291.1
pathological drunkenness	291.4
Alcohol-related psychoses	
hallucinosis	291.3
jealousy	291.5
mania	291.9
paranoia	291.5
psychosis NOS	291.9
Alcohol withdrawal states	
delirium tremens	291.0
other	291.8
Conduct disorders	
adjustment reaction	309.3/309.4
disturbance of conduct	
compulsive	312.2
mixed (emotions)	312.3
socialized	312.1
unsocialized	312.0

*This should be used as an *index* to ICD-9 and not as a *substitute* for it.

Conduct disorders (continued)	
frontal lobe syndrome	310.0
personality disorder	
explosive	301.3
sociopathic	301.7
Dementia	
alcoholic	291.2
depressed type	290.2
paranoid type	290.2
presenile type	290.1
simple type	290.0
with acute confusional state	290.3
multi-infarct	290.4
other	290.8
other – conditions classified elsewhere	294.1
Depressive disorders	
acute (depressive) reaction to stress	308.0
affective personality disorder	301.1
brief depressive reaction	309.0
depressive disorder NEC	311
manic-depressive psychosis, circular depressed	296.3
manic-depressive psychosis, circular, mixed	296.4
manic-depressive psychosis, depressed	296.1
neurotic depression	300.4
prolonged depressive reaction	309.1
reactive depressive psychosis	298.0
rebound depression following mania	296.8
schizoaffective psychosis	295.7
senile dementia, depressed type	290.2
Drug-related disorders	
dependence	304
non-dependent abuse	305
Drug-related psychoses	
acute confusional state	293.0
other	292.8
paranoid and/or hallucinatory state	292.1
pathological intoxication	292.2
subacute confusional state	293.1
unspecified	292.9
Drug withdrawal states	292.0

Intoxication	
alcohol	305.0
drug	305.2–305.9
pathological	
alcohol	291.4
drug	292.2
Mania	
alcoholic	291.9
manic-depressive psychosis	296.0/296.2/296.4
mixed paranoid and affective organic psychosis	294.8
reactive excitative psychosis	298.1
Neurosis	
anxiety	300.0
depersonalization	300.6
depressive	300.4
hypochondriacal	300.7
hysterical	300.1
neurasthenia	300.5
obsessive-compulsive	300.3
other	300.8
phobic	300.2
Organic psychoses	
(see also Alcohol-related psychoses, Dementia, Drug-related psychoses).	
acute confusional state	293.0
epileptic psychosis NOS	294.8
mixed paranoid and affective	294.8
subacute confusional state	293.1
Paranoid psychoses	
(excluding schizophrenia – qv).	
acute paranoid reaction	298.3
alcoholic paranoia	291.5
drug-induced	292.1
induced psychosis	297.3
mixed paranoid and affective organic	294.8
other	297.8
paranoia	297.1
paranoid state, simple	297.0
paraphrenia	297.2
psychogenic	298.4
senile dementia, paranoid type	290.2

Personality disorders	
affective	301.1
asocial	301.7
asthenic	301.6
explosive	301.3
frontal lobe syndrome	310.0
hysterical	301.5
other	301.8
paranoid	301.0
post-traumatic personality change	310.1
schizoid	301.2
sociopathic	301.7
unspecified	301.9
Reactive disorders, psychotic	
acute paranoid reaction	298.3
confusion, reactive	298.2
depressive (reactive) psychosis	298.0
excitative reactive psychosis	298.1
hysterical psychosis	298.8
psychogenic paranoid psychosis	298.4
psychogenic stupor	298.8
Reactive disorders, non-psychotic	
acute reactions to stress	308
adjustment reactions	309
depressive reaction (neurosis)	300.4
Schizophrenia	
acute (undifferentiated)	295.8
acute schizophrenic episode	295.4
catatonic	295.2
hebephrenic	295.1
latent	295.5
other	295.8
paranoid	295.3
residual	295.6
schizoaffective	295.7
simple	295.0
unspecified	295.9

Index